CASE STUDIES
IN LEFT AND RIGHT
HEMISPHERIC FUNCTIONING

CASE STUDIES
IN LEFT AND RIGHT
HEMISPHERIC FUNCTIONING

By

JACK L. FADELY

*Associate Professor of Special Education
and Educational Psychology
College of Education
Butler University
Indianapolis, Indiana*

and

VIRGINIA N. HOSLER

*Diagnostic Learning Center
Peoria Public Schools
Peoria, Illinois*

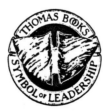

CHARLES C THOMAS • PUBLISHER
Springfield • Illinois • U.S.A.

Published and Distributed Throughout the World by

CHARLES C THOMAS • PUBLISHER

2600 South First Street

Springfield, Illinois, 62717, U.S.A.

© *1983 by* CHARLES C THOMAS • PUBLISHER

ISBN 0-398-04792-8

Library of Congress Catalog Card Number: 82-19212

Printed in the United States of America

I-R-1

Library of Congress Cataloging in Publication Data

Fadely, Jack L., 1934–
    Case studies in left and right hemispheric functioning.

    Bibliography: p.
    Includes index.
    1. Left and right (Psychology) 2. Learning, Psychology of.
3. Educational psychology. I. Hosler, Virginia N., 1943–   .
II. Title. [DNLM: 1. Laterality – Case studies. 2. Learning –
In infancy and childhood – Case studies. 3. Learning – Physi-
ology – Case studies. 4. Teaching – Methods – Case studies.
WL 335 F144c]
BF723.L25F33   1983   370.15'23   82-19212
ISBN 0-398-04792-8

INTRODUCTION

THE decade of the 1980s opened with an increasing concern in the educational field for the individual student and for the discouragingly high number of illiterate adults in the United States. These two concerns are not unassociated, but neither are they as closely related as one might assume. It could be thought, by a historian, that concern for the level of illiteracy marked the beginning of an increased concern for understanding the needs of the individual student. This is not the case, although educators are well aware of both concerns during this decade. In education we find ourselves pressured by society for an increased accountability in teaching at a time when cutbacks in federal funds, difficulties in obtaining local funds, and a host of additional factors are all making it difficult to really reach the individual. Yet, within the field of education, many newer theories of instruction and individualization are being offered to schools daily to assist in helping every child learn. The problem will become, as it already has, how to deliver new technology to teachers in the classroom. It was once said that it took twenty-five years for a new technology in teaching to reach the majority of classrooms across the country. That is no longer true, but certainly new technology is still slow in coming to the local classroom teacher who, too often, has little choice in the materials she will use or the number of students she must teach.

The university has long been the means by which teachers have upgraded their skills and learned of new technology. Today teachers are neither prone, nor can they afford in either time or money, to return to the college classroom. Further, it must be questioned if this is the best way to upgrade a teacher's skills. Universities, no less than local schools, are bound by tradition and bureaucracy, and are slow to change themselves. Until recently the university had a corner on the market for supplying schools with trained teachers and the availability of training for those already teaching. But today the pace of change in both understanding children, and how to teach, has outdistanced the university's capacity to communicate such changes via teacher training. Education has become big business, and the field of business has found a profit in providing new technology to schools directly. The most significant example is the microcomputer which is presently being sold directly to schools, along with hardware and software that often are beyond the competency or knowledge of most university teacher trainers.

But as important as hardware and software may be, along with other newer means of providing instruction to children, another field has much to offer that will be significant in the management of computer instruction. The field of child development, including the collective efforts of child psychologists, neurologists, and educational psychologists, is opening up entirely new ways of looking at children and how they learn. This additional body of knowledge is promising to change forever our concepts of learning, and in the process much of the newer theory of computer education will have to be altered to accommodate this information. With all of this occurring outside of the classroom, the teacher is caught in an ever widening gap between her knowledge and that available to her.

Within the field of child development, one of the many theories that has been developing in recent years is that of the effects of brain lateralization on learning. At first it has the flavor of another esoteric concept that will have little to do with the everyday practice of teaching. As it turns out, it has great relevance, and is part of a range of newer concepts about teaching in which the concern is how children learn and, more specifically, how to determine how each child should be taught to maximize his likelihood of learning. The lateralization theory is but one of these newer approaches, but it is a significant one which is being popularized through the notion of right and left brain learning.

This book is a third generation book in the field of brain lateralization and learning. The first book by the authors, *Understanding the Alpha Child at Home and at School*, provided basic introductory information on how specific differences in left and right brain function affects how children learn. That book also pointed out how teaching methodology has to be adapted to children relative to their particular organization in brain lateralization. Following that book, the authors also published *Holistic Mental Health for Tomorrow's Children*, which took the brain lateralization theory a step further, and discussed it in relation to personality and behavior. One of the difficulties encountered when these first two books were used with classroom teachers was the difficulty teachers had in applying the concepts to children. This book, *Case Studies in Left and Right Hemispheric Functioning*, alleviates that difficulty by providing teachers and psychologists with case studies which bring the theory directly into the classroom through concrete examples.

The present book is designed to be easily read and understood by classroom teachers and others concerned with individualization of instruction.

CONTENTS

CASE STUDIES
IN LEFT AND RIGHT
HEMISPHERIC FUNCTIONING

Chapter 1
LEFT AND RIGHT HEMISPHERIC
BRAIN THEORY

IT was sometime near the middle of the 1970s that Robert Ornstein published his book on right and left hemispheric brain function and launched, almost unnoticed at the time, a movement that began to grow in separate parts of this country and others. Many neurologists and psychoneurologists were investigating the mysteries of the right hemisphere, most being concerned with perception, various problems in epilepsy and other cerebral dysfunctions, including brain injury and biochemical factors in brain function. From many points within the medical and psychological professions, individuals were beginning to see new perspectives on the so-called "minor" hemisphere and yet, at that point in the early 1970s little had been synthesized. Dimond and Beaumont published a book in England in 1974 entitled *Hemispheric Function in the Human Brain*, which brought together research from a broad front completed in recent years. The book was picked up by Halsted Press of Wiley & Sons but, most regretfully, by the late 1970s was out of print. Sir Karl Popper and Sir John Eccles contributed their book, *The Self and Its Brain*, during the same period. During the 1970s other books by capable professionals also appeared that investigated the hemispheric relationship and the consequences of cerebral specialization on both learning and behavior. Within professional circles there was much interest and controversy about the whole phenomenon of left and right hemispheric function. Finally, the silent partner to the major and language hemisphere had been discovered it seemed, and new theories were being developed amidst much excitement and debate.

3

But it was not until the early 1980s that the laboratories of neurology and psychology began to yield information that could be picked up by the public, which is always eager for some new theory on how we think and why we act as we do. It was time to "popularize" hemisphericity and the whole left and right brain theory. The first gleams of enlightenment popped up in psychological journals and educational literature with such articles as "Right Brained Kids in Left Brained Schools," and "How to Teach the Right Side of the Brain." In the first two years of the 1980s more than ten major books have appeared in both the textbook and trade market that purport to inform the public and professional alike about the wonders of the right-left brain theory and its importance to children and adults. The final burst of excitement is best illustrated by a Volvo® commercial in a major magazine in which the qualities of the Volvo were outlined on one page for your left brain and on the other page for your right brain. Right brain theory has definitely made the popular market.

Our own book, *Understanding the Alpha Child at Home and at School*, published by Charles C Thomas, Publishers, in 1979, was the result of clinical research with children beginning in the early part of 1973. It was not a popular trade book though the title might have implied as much. It was in our minds an attempt to synthesize our own efforts and available research into a book that teachers and psychologists could use as an introduction to the concept of hemispheric specialization in relation to behavior and learning. We tried to take a stand between neurological theory and education in an attempt to give some practical application to concepts about hemispheric specialization.

The book has been used with several hundred graduate students in education and psychology over the years since its publication, and the authors found that they had overestimated those students. It would be nice to say that the ability of such students and professionals to comprehend the concept had been underestimated, but, unfortunately their ability to synthesize new information had been overestimated. In presenting the material to professionals two major problems were initially encountered: the often rigid mind set that professionals have about information within their field; and the difficulties that most professionals have in using their "right brain" capacity to see holistic concepts instead of "left brain" digital and bit information. They understood the parts but could not see the whole. Fortunately, the problem was resolved through the use of case studies which the authors had in abundance from over ten years of work with children and adults who displayed unusual hemispheric balance.

The authors followed the first book with another, *Holistic Mental Health for Tomorrow's Children*, which applied the theory to mental health and personality of children in schools. That book seemed to be more easily assimilated by the students, but again case studies were needed to truly demonstrate the nature and extent of hemispheric effects on behavior and learning. It was that experience that prompted the writing of this third book, which, as far as we have found in the proliferation of new popular and professional books in the area, takes a step beyond most books and actually demonstrates the practicalities and difficulties of applying the hemispheric concepts.

The present book is written primarily for those professionals who have an interest in the concept and have read or worked within the area. Yet, many professionals who have not read other material will surely find their way to this book; and so we find ourselves needing to explain the theory on one hand and to apply that information on the other. For those with some background in the area we must beg their patience at times as we retrace some of our earlier discussions in other works. Perhaps, this will also assist in giving all of us a common background to better understand the cases discussed.

The first problem which may confront us is the unwise choice we originally made in calling the first book *The Alpha Child*, instead of simply left and right hemispheric brain theory with children. One of our concerns in the first book was that many writers would take the popular approach and treat the theory as some new and mysterious finding that would reveal yet another panacea for education and psychology. We were right, as the market is now revealing. Our own book was perhaps little better than the rest, because we not only seemed to be moving on to a new concept but also creating a new sort of special child as well. And yet, we do not apologize for our approach, because it has great importance as will be seen in the coming studies. Where most authors have attempted to address the whole of the concern for right and left brain function, we have been concerned for children who demonstrate a particular aspect of the theory. It is true that today's schools do not emphasize and assist children in learning to exercise the naturalistic and holistic abilities normally associated with right hemispheric function, but our concern was not for that general issue. We were concerned with those children who demonstrate dominant right hemispheric function to the detriment of developing capable language function. The total human being is the fortunate individual who exhibits competence in both language and nonverbal or naturalistic thought. Barring that level of competence the individual who demonstrates at least high competence in language function is a lucky individual for he can succeed in school and society. But our concern is for that unlucky child who demonstrates average or below average language capacity and yet high levels of competence in nonverbal function. The naturalistic child with high competence in nonverbal function lives on an alien planet for he has little in common with either the schools or society. This is our alpha child. These are the children that we had discovered and worked with in the last decade that brought us through the back door to the whole hemispheric concept. Like the alpha child we did it backwards. If people have difficulty understanding the concept of hemisphericity they are certain to miss totally the notion of the "right" and naturalistic child. He is being cast off as emotionally disturbed, learning disabled, or socially maladjusted, although he is essentially normal except his being a mirror image of the typical high language and uncreative child that schools and society love so much.

The Hemisphericity Movement in Education

While much of the popular literature presently refers to the specialization of function in the hemispheres as left and right brain theory, we prefer to call the phenomenon "hemisphericity" and will use that term throughout our discussions here. The movement in education is primarily being recognized as having relevance to school curriculum and the highly verbal nature of school instruction. The focus of much of the concern in education is how to increase and improve those aspects of the curriculum that teach and develop nonverbal or creative aspects of individual learning. This interest is taking several directions and much of it rides more on a sort of "enthusiasm for creative behavior" rather than the more serious and important aspects of the concept.

In order to understand the current movement and the more important aspects that may fail to be recognized, a moment should be spent reviewing the overall concept. (A more detailed discussion of the concept can be found in our earlier books or other literature on the subject should the reader have such interest.) We will touch on many of the problems in understanding hemisphericity in the practical setting when working with children as we proceed through the case studies.

There is a simplistic viewpoint, shared primarily by educators unfamiliar with neurological function and child development, which we will present first and then add some comments which should be presented in light of that simpler notion. The study of brain function, while quite old, has accelerated in recent years, but much of the literature on the brain still available does not take into account many of the more recent findings.

Dr. William Penfield, a neurosurgeon, wrote eloquently, in a book called *Mysteries of the Mind*, about his long interest in "mapping" areas of the brain. He was perhaps one of the major pioneers of the study of brain function and hemisphericity. Localizing specific areas of neuro-function occupied the work of neurologists throughout the first part of this century. The two hemispheres of the brain contained major divisions, including the visual areas at the rear, sensory and motor areas toward the middle, and the frontal and temporal lobes at the front and sides. Much of the tissue in the rear and middle of the hemispheres is genetically committed tissue, that is, it comes at birth with more or less programmed functions to perform. The areas of interest in hemisphericity are primarily those in the prefrontal and frontal lobes and the temporal lobes at the side of the frontal portion of each hemisphere. (See Figure 1.) The frontal lobes are extensive tissue areas that are to a large degree unprogrammed at birth and are receptive to the effects of environment on their development during the first years of life.

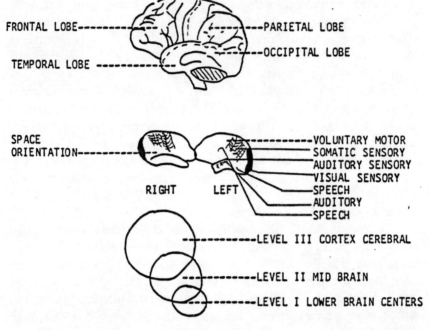

Figure 1. Various areas of functioning in central nervous system.

The left hemisphere, specifically areas around the temporal lobes of that hemisphere, demonstrates significant anatomical differences from the same areas in the right hemisphere. These areas are the sites of language function including speech, recognition of sounds used for language, auditory memory and other language-related abilities. In most human brains this anatomical difference exists, and due to the importance of language as the symbol system in learning and communication, this hemisphere has traditionally been regarded as the "major" hemisphere with the right hemisphere designated as the "minor" hemisphere. Early damage to the left hemisphere language areas can sometimes be compensated for by the similar areas in the right hemisphere. Normally, however, the same temporal areas in the right hemisphere appear to be specialized to process spatial information as opposed to language.

The frontal lobes of both hemispheres appear to process information concerning foresight and synthesis of various data. The corpus callosum, which connects the two hemispheres, is a massive area of tissue providing a communication and integrative function for information between the two hemispheres. Much of the earlier information concerning the specialization of the two hemispheres was obtained from brain-damaged patients or from patients suffering from epilepsy, which was relieved at times through cutting the corpus callosum. These "split-brain" patients were then studied, yielding information about the effects of preventing the exchange between the two hemispheres.

It was found that although both hemispheres received information from all sensory inputs, each hemisphere appeared to specialize in synthesizing either language or spatial information. Some authors have compared the structure of neuronic tissue in each hemisphere to computers. (It should be remembered, however, that when we speak of hemispheric specialization we are primarily referring only to the temporal and frontal lobes.) The language-based structure of the left hemisphere appears to organize itself to synthesize information into "bits" or, in comparison to computers, into "digital" data. The right hemisphere tissue, conversely, appears to organize information in a very different way and one might refuse the use of the word "organize" altogether. The right hemisphere appears to process information through a more "holistic" or total manner utilizing primarily nonverbal sensory data. For example, in young infants it was found the EEG responses to verbal and nonverbal information which was auditory in nature diffused in the two hemispheres. When phonetic sounds were played the left hemisphere responded in an organized manner while the right tended to emit nonresponsive patterns. But when nonphonetic sounds such as whistles, horns, or animal noises were played the right hemisphere became active with the left becoming inactive. This demonstrated that the two hemispheres were already responding in a specialized way during the first few days of life. The right hemisphere then appears to respond to spatial and nonverbal information, making it more of an analog computer.

A simple, perhaps too simple at this point, example of the integrative and specializing relation between the analog and digital computers in our head can be seen in reading or writing. When one reads, the right hemisphere recognizes and discriminates visual form and space which is then digitalized by the left hemisphere into sounds and eventually words. This is not the only way the brain can read, as we will see later, but the example illustrates how in many behaviors the specialization of the two hemispheres is important in an integrated and complex learning task. Conversely, when a child is daydreaming, building a block tower, or listening to music, the right hemisphere plays the primary role in behavior. When the child is talking or listening to directions from the teacher the left hemisphere comes into play as the dominant mode of controlling consciousness or concentration. With this general overview let us now look at the specific functions attributed to each hemisphere. But always remember that both hemispheres receive the same information and that there is always a combination of specialization and yet alteration of specific function between and within the two hemispheres.

The Left Hemispheric Functions

1. Recognition and control of speech.
2. Reception, storage, and synthesis of verbal-auditory data.
3. Serialization of data and sequential organization of verbal information.
4. Comprehension and utilization of temporal (time) memory and behavior.

These functions have been well established in neurological literature as located within left hemispheric specialization. There are language functions in the right hemisphere also but these are minor in comparison to the major role of the left hemisphere. Being educators and having observed children, the authors realized that if the foregoing functions were left hemispheric then certain other functions had to be inferred. For example, social values and concepts and basically abstract and verbal functions would also be implicated in left hemispheric function. On that basis then the following functions are also attributed to the left hemisphere by the authors, although neurological research would not usually approach these learning and behavioral functions.

5. Logical and rational behavior, i.e. doing something according to a language-based concept or learned verbal orientation.
6. Socialized values, i.e. understanding and following the abstract social values of the culture.
7. Social competition and behavior relating to evaluating self according to a social doctrine or religious value.
8. Higher mathematical skills that involve formulization and time-space concepts, particularly in abstract form.
9. Perception of self in relation to concepts of time and sequence of events.

The Right Hemispheric Functions

1. Recognition of nonverbal auditory information and minor comprehension of language.
2. Recognition and manipulation of form and shapes, form-space relationships, behaviors of objects and people, and meaning in nonverbal information, i.e. the smile or threat face.
3. Perceptual gestalt, seeing the whole of a thing, and awareness of the totality of a perceptual object.
4. Creative and artistic skills, producing images and altering sensory data into new forms — creativity.
5. Recognition and synthesis of musical perception, rhythm and movement patterns in music.
6. Integration and execution of complex gross and fine motor movements, i.e. the surgeon operating or the football player passing the ball during the game.
7. Intuitiveness and insight — Recognition of meaning within nonverbal behavior and activity about us — appreciation of the flight of a bird or the purpose of mechanical functions.
8. Concrete math functions, simple calculations.
9. Artistic abilities and appreciation.

These overall functions have been ascribed by various researchers to the left and right hemispheres. It can be seen how an individual may at times utilize primarily information from one hemisphere or the other depending upon the specific behaviors that are under concentration.

In reviewing these functions several important factors come to light in working with and understanding children within the educational setting. The example of reading illustrates that both spatial and verbal functions must be developed. But there are several general developmental principles that must also be understood.

1. Development of cerebral competency moves from sensory experience to language abstraction.

The young infant does not talk and does not initially use much language in that the first year is occupied with learning to control and use the body (sensorimotor structure.) The right hemisphere is critical in early movement and sensorimotor development; therefore we postulate that during the first years the right hemisphere is the dominant hemisphere and directs the early learning of the child. As movement patterns are established and increasing kinesthetic, tactile, taste, smell, visual, and nonverbal information is learned, then left hemispheric function comes into play to name, categorize, label, and organize experience into an abstraction. In essence, language follows experience during the first few years and then eventually, with increased cognitive development, the left hemisphere becomes dominant. This explains why experiential-based curriculum programs make more sense for younger children.

2. Affectual or emotional components of consciousness are most closely tied to right hemispheric function.

The early bonding and attachment of the infant to his mother is accomplished through tactile and kinesthetic sensory data. This data is processed and synthesized most critically within the right hemisphere. Therefore, the feeling components of human relationships are most likely tied more critically to right hemispheric function than to the more rational and abstract processes in the left hemisphere. We tell someone we love them through the left hemisphere but the love exists in the right hemisphere.

We like to refer to the left hemisphere as the "socialized" mind and the right hemisphere as the "naturalistic" mind. It becomes obvious that curiosity, emotions, play, fantasy, and for that matter the very nature of childhood are contained within the impulsive and sensitive right or naturalized hemisphere. Childhood is lost as the left hemisphere and cultural values come to dominate the child's consciousness. But then so are creative abilities such as the ability to dream and imagine. This is the point upon which much of the current left and right hemisphere literature in educational areas is being focused. This is a point upon which we elaborate to some length in our book, *Holistic Mental Health for Tomorrow's Children.*

Thus far then, education has not focused upon helping children learn to continue to use their creative abilities, to nurture and develop the naturalistic hemisphere. This fact is one that needs to be emphasized in education and at home. But, this emphasis is missing important massive areas of the theory and it is toward those areas that much of our discussion will focus throughout the book. It is our concern that educators will only understand the one aspect and miss, in our estimation, the truly comprehensive and far-reaching implications of the whole theory. After all it seems easier to focus on the more simplistic aspects of a new theory. That is the problem we have run into in attempting to assist educators and psychologists during our lectures and work.

This book is written with as little clinical terminology as possible to make it readable and understandable to educators and psychologists. Educators, we find, tend to look for simpler solutions and notions about how children learn while too often psychologists tend to deal with the bits and pieces of the data yielded from their tests and miss the problem altogether. We are not being disrespectful to either group but, as will be seen in the case study analysis, neither approach usually yields practical help for the child. We trust that the more clinically minded of our readers can utilize the data presented should they desire a more in-depth look at the information. But, as a consequence of the problem educators and psychologists have had in understanding our earlier work, we will make every attempt to look at these cases and the theory from a learning and practical standpoint. Further, we work with children every day and our own interest lies in the practical aspects of the theory and not the more profound implications of brain function and neurology. From the direction that much of the literature is moving, however, we feel there is a desperate need to present an overall and holistic viewpoint of the ramifications of hemispheric function in relation to personality and learning. No other authors at this point have approached the theory from a case study point of view.

Learning Disabilities and Hemisphericity

In *Understanding the Alpha Child at Home and School* we touched often on the probability that the entire field of learning disabilities was in need of evaluation, and from our experience in schools with learning disabled children, it has become apparent that the rampaging irrationality about learning disabilities that has so gripped schools in the last fifteen years must somehow be brought under control. At the past rate of diagnosis it would appear that many school systems will have all of their children except the very brightest in classes for the learning disabled. The whole concept of developmental deficit is mostly in error and has resulted in too many children who demonstrated no significant neurological or developmental disorders being placed in classes for the learning disabled. Many parents have lovingly embraced the learning disabilities concept to explain failing children and yet it has not really helped much. There seems to always be another disability discovered or created by someone. Dyslexic children run happily down every school corridor, and hyperactive children will soon surely form their own union for theirs is one of the fastest growing number in the country. Yet, working with learning disabled children and the general theory of child development and hemisphericity we have come to know that the majority of learning disabilities are not in the child at all but in the lack of competent instruction in our schools. The greatest single cause of dyslexia is poor instruction; and hyperactivity, aside from the many nutritional and metabolic cases, must be laid primarily at the feet of poor parenting (as we discussed in *Understanding the Alpha Child at Home and School*).

Yet, we do not wish to write a book about the irrationality and outright criminality of learning disabilities pushers. We want to utilize hemispheric theory to help parents and teachers learn that many children are not disabled. Many of the children who seem to have a learning disability in reality have a developmental difference based in the peculiarities of how the central nervous system may develop in any specific child. Further, these developmental differences can be compensated for or resolved through effective instruction or behavioral therapy and never need be called or labeled a disability. The whole field of learning disabilities has been terribly important, however, in bringing teachers to the realization that children must be understood within their own special ways of learning. The next step will be for teachers to forget learning disabilities and simply look at the marvelous ways that children learn and adapt teaching methods to fit their needs. That is part of what we want to demonstrate through our case studies because we have seen literally thousands of children who had personality and learning difficulties reach successful adjustment and learning through normal classroom effort once everyone understood something about how they learn. This book then, will be of great importance to those who cherish and engulf themselves in the disabilities phenomenon, because hopefully it will assist them in looking at their children in a way other than as damaged wayfarers who need treatment.

Pseudo-Psychological Phenomenon: Merlin the Psychologist

Psychologists do much good work. As one psychologist stated after a small child ran through his freshly cemented patio, "I highly recommend children in the abstract but not in the concrete." We highly recommend school psychologists to the children. We hope that is taken in the good humor of its presentation. And we must qualify that statement too, for we mean developmental and school psychologists and not clinical psychologists.

It has been with some amusement in the last two or three years that we have reviewed presenters' titles at school psychology seminars and conferences. As in the learning disabilities field, psychologists have suddenly leaped upon the hemisphericity phenomenon and are now intensely "working" with the theory. As one might expect, psychologists do not simply present left and right brain approaches to learning, as do the learning disabilities people, but rather they come up with such titles as "Psychoneurological Correlates in Learning Disabilities." Suddenly school psychologists have become psychoneurologists and are utilizing the hemisphericity movement to develop some respect for their daily task of administering Binets and WISCs to unsuspecting children in the schools. Suddenly Billy no longer has a learning disability but hemispheric competition or dysfunction. That should really "wow" the parents and create another national organization for parents. It will be called Association for Parents of Children with Hemispheric Peculiarities, perhaps.

But while we may poke fun at our tendency to label and create titles and movements, we do recognize that most parents, teachers, and psychologists are dedicated and concerned individuals who want somehow to help children sort it all out. We are no less to blame than any others, and yet our work with children and parents has constantly humbled us because the final answer is never quite there. What we have learned from the hemispheric theory is that there are other ways to look at children than simply making an analysis of their deficits. We can learn to understand the realities of child development in more detail and find ways to help children as they are. So we ask ourselves and the theory makers to show us a child and tell us how the theory works for this child here, today, in this classroom. That is the sort of confrontation we have had in our graduate classes and in the classroom of the teacher who must work with the real child in front of her. The theory can be of great assistance to both parents and teachers, if we can apply it and understand in a holistic manner what all of our data mean. It will not help us though to make up a lot of new titles or present ourselves as pseudo-psychoneurologists. Let us throw out our need for recognition and get the task done.

Hemisphericity in Curriculum Planning

In our discussions here it should become obvious that much of what can be learned from hemisphericity can be applied not only to special children but to the general curriculum for all children as well. But the present trend is toward focusing on the stimulation of high function on the naturalistic and creative aspects of the child's development. That, as we have mentioned, is shortsighted and does not utilize the more valuable aspects of what is being learned from the general theory.

The critical aspects of the hemisphericity theory are those that deal with general concepts of how the central nervous system develops and functions and which point to specific ways in which children should be taught. It is common today, in some areas of education, to speak of visual and auditory learners and yet, too often, it is a misnomer to call a child a visual or auditory learner for almost always he is both. Yet, we develop methods to teach the visual learner and the auditory learner differently. The brain simply does not function in one major modality when processing complex information, whether it is primarily verbal or spatial. It is the *integration* of hemispheric function that provides the key to understanding how a child learns.

School curriculum is not mathematics or language arts. These are specific and yet complex skills which accomplish something far more important. They allow the child to learn how to learn. It is what a child learns, what he is capable of feeling and accomplishing in becoming a whole person that makes of schools more than numbers or letters. We can help the child learn the critical things without his being able to add numbers or read letters. We teach him numbers and letters that he will also be able to learn without our help. The most important element in hemispheric theory is to come to understand not how to merely teach letters or numbers but to understand how the child "thinks," to understand how he "solves" problems, "creates" ideas, and learns to communicate with others. Hemispheric theory then should not be, as it is already becoming, simply another trick in our teaching bag to help the child learn to read. That is important, but school curriculum will best be served when we understand child development well enough that we can "see" how children think. That will be one of our goals in the coming discussions.

The Holistic Matrix Within Child Development

It would be just as appropriate to say the "holy matrix" in child development. Within the interaction of biological structures of the human body arises an entity that is less physical than metaphysical, an organizing energy that has no form and no known basis, a thing called self, a thing we know as "the child." This phenomenon that we call a person is a consciousness that seems more to accompany its physical self than to be part of it. One should never, we are told, mix feelings and science. We have tried to do that and found it boring. Without feelings one does not work with children. We have been told as teachers and psychologists that we should remain objective with children who are our charges. To that we say rubbish! Every child who walks through our clinic door or into our classroom is at once a living being for whom we are accepting responsibility. If we cannot tolerate the responsibility then, as Truman said, "If you can't take the heat, get out of the kitchen!" We find it hard to maintain an ethical and professional relationship with a four-year-old who is throwing ice at us from his McDonald's Coke® cup now drained of its nectar. We find it difficult to remain objective when a ten-year-old first grader discovers he can read after all, if we let him give up phonetics. When you test, teach, or accept a child into your world to share his thoughts you are stuck and whether you want the responsibility or not you have it. . .for life.

We never forget and neither do the children or their parents. This child before us whom we are going to teach or test has come there in good faith that we have something to offer him in the way of making things a little better for him. Mechanics are lucky, they take a part off, replace it, and put on the new part. It is all over and no one need start a relationship. The child's part cannot be replaced, and most often it does not need to be, if we can just figure out how to help the child make it work. Failing that we try · to help him learn to do what the rest of us do with parts that do not work too well. Either way the child can win.

A child is always becoming himself. He is never complete, and the sooner we all learn that, the easier it will be to look at the whole child and not just his problem. We do not work with children simply to "fix" something that is wrong. We help children learn how to get to the next place they want to go or where we think they ought to be going. That, interestingly enough, is part of what hemisphericity can teach us. We are not trying to learn something special about the brain, we are learning about the child who happens to be part of that brain.

Children develop as whole units and within the unit are special parts that all have to work together, including motor functions, visual and perceptual functions, space, time, and words, thoughts, dreams, and concerns. Somehow all of this has to come together to make sense to the child.

In our coming discussion we will use the theory of hemisphericity as but another unifying concept in learning how to understand the whole of children and how they learn. Somehow we *must* get that message across to those who read this book. Hemisphericity is a theory about neurological function, but in essence it is but another way of looking at the whole issue of how children develop. Unless it is integrated into what little we have already learned it will become another "fad" that will be lost when the next trick is invented. Each new theory is but another block, another piece, in the complex puzzle of consciousness and personal being. The more we learn the more likely we will be able to help our children toward a more holistic understanding of both themselves and life. If that sounds a bit grandiose then give us something more important to do.

Chapter 2
THE BASIC CONSTRUCTS OF
LEFT AND RIGHT
HEMISPHERIC FUNCTIONING

THE basis upon which much of the hemispheric theory rests is that of specialization of certain functions of perception, language, spatial abilities, memory, and cognitive activities into one or the other hemisphere. Names such as Sperry, Penfield, Ornstein, Geschmind, Trevarthen, Gazzinga, Levy, and Dimond are but a few of the distinguished professionals who have contributed much to the emerging theory of hemispheric function. These researchers and so many others are unfamiliar to most educators and perhaps most school psychologists. We will not dwell on the many studies that are available concerning specific aspects of hemispericity in this presentation. Ours is not an attempt to persuade the reader that such research exists or that it is in need of our own summary or analysis. That we have done to some degree in other work. For the psychologist who wishes to delve further into the specificity of research techniques or data a rather lengthy bibliography appears at the end of the book. For the teacher or practitioner in the field of education and psychology we wish, rather, to present a summary of the various notions that have been gleaned from the research and give the reader some idea of basic principles based on that research which seem to apply to working directly with children. There are several general constructs that we will utilize from the research and we are certain to recognize that to a large degree our constructs probably have been less available to the other researchers than have specific constructs about left and right field visual-brain operations, for

20

example. These basic constructs have come from the researchers and have been applied with children, resulting in practical and working methodology in understanding or helping children learn and adjust.

1. The brain, at birth, presents a degree of plasticity that allows it to form neurological structures appropriate to the demands placed upon it by the particular environment within which it finds itself.

2. Human intelligence, the ability of the brain to adapt and develop behavioral responses to the environment, is founded first in the integrities provided by genetics and secondly in the competence of the environment to provide stimulation appropriate to mental growth.

3. The hemispheres of the brain tend to specialize certain functions into the left or right hemisphere, although both hemispheres receive the same sensory information. In the main, both hemispheres at birth have somewhat similar potential to develop in all learning areas.

4. The left hemisphere is anatomically structured at birth to process and develop functions related to language although the right also has such facilities. If all proceeds normally, the language areas of the left hemisphere acquire language function, with spatial integration becoming an essential specialization of the right hemisphere.

5. The corpus callosum provides an interhemispheric route of exchanging sensory data and processed data from either hemisphere to the other. This communication link also makes it possible for each hemisphere to "know" of the activities of its associate, although it may not actually perform the processing activity of the other hemisphere.

6. Specialization of certain functions within each hemisphere is called lateralization and, in various individuals, may be accomplished to a greater or lesser degree, resulting in a wide variance of any individual to process information in the same way. There appear to be sexual differences relative to degree and nature of lateralization.

7. The concept of mature intelligence can be roughly divided into intellectual functions in verbal and spatial areas, and these

are usually best understood within the diagnostic structure of the WISC-R Intelligence Test.

8. The intelligence score represents, rather than a measure of some innate ability, the sum total of a child's abilities from genetic and environmental influences and his ability to utilize those competencies. Increased or decreased competency in a specific function or an entire cluster of functions, i.e. verbal or spatial, can be affected by environment.

9. Competence within a specific hemisphere's specialty may be thought of as hemispheric efficiency, or competence, and is a measure of efficiency in function. Wide disparities between the levels of competence between the two hemispheres can dramatically alter the learning and behavioral style of the individual.

10. The foundations of personality can be directly related to hemispheric functions and competence just as hemispheric competence can be affected by mental health.

11. Lateralization of functions into the left hemisphere, digital and sequential language based, and the right hemisphere, holistic and analogous toward creative function, produces a greater potentiality in competence than either alone or the sum total of the individual parts. This principle allows then that the greatest human potential is not in either verbal or spatial but in the integrative functions.

12. Consciousness both in its quality and quantity of function is dependent upon the development of specialized qualities in the two hemispheres. Learning and processing information in an integrated way produces a greater awareness of self and the ability to perceive both subjective and objective experience more effectively.

13. Consciousness in conventional modes is accomplished within the functions of the left hemispheric competence while intuition and transcendence in thought is accomplished through the holistic modes of right hemispheric thought.

14. Naturalistic thought is basic to all living things and is combined with self-consciousness first through right hemispheric development. Left hemispheric dominance is achieved through the eventual abstracting functions of socialized and left hemispheric development.

15. Naturalistic thought tends to be nondirectional, although it often tends toward right-left organization as in left-handed children due to the sensory orientation of right hemispheric organization.

16. Socialized thought tends to be directional toward left-right organization and produces an orientation typical of right-handed people.

17. The natural tendency is for left hemispheric dominance and language superiority over naturalistic organization.

18. The relationship of cerebral dominance to hand, eye, ear, and foot dominance tends to be one of lateral organization, that is, left hemispheric dominance, right-handedness, right ear and footedness, and right visual dominance.

19. Either hemisphere can control either motor side, although normally the hand is controlled by the opposite hemisphere.

20. Poor establishment of cerebral dominance, hand dominance, or visual-hand dominance can create disorganization in the spatial function of the child.

The reader, upon reviewing these general constructs, can begin to appreciate the complexity of understanding hemisphericity. The implications of the research, stated here in these constructs, are probably enough to frighten even the bravest of teachers away from the notion. It is easy to see why one clings to a simple notion that there is a left and right brain after attempting to read the research studies, each dealing with minute parts of specific perceptual, language, or behavioral function.

Each of these constructs will be utilized in understanding the specific educational and emotional needs of the children in the case studies and, although it would appear remote at this point, it all will become clearer with the analysis of the cases. The reader must bear with us and trust that these constructs can be turned into practical techniques for understanding and teaching children. But it should be obvious here that we are talking about far more than simply a theory of right and left brain function. We are, in reality, discussing an overview of the general integrative functions in child development and learning.

Diagnosis of Hemisphericity: Practical and Theoretical

How does one go about diagnosing hemisphericity? First, let us state that one does not diagnose hemisphericity and that is one of the problems we see beginning in the current interest of psychologists in the hemispheric concept. Many professionals are approaching the theory from a strictly "neuroplumbing" viewpoint, meaning that the psychologist is looking at all of this as if it were an exercise in psychoneurology; unfortunately that approach will only help us discover deficits, lesions, damage, and perhaps a syndrome or two. For example, we can tell a teacher that the child has poor reticular stimulation of cortical functions resulting in lowered organizational ability, or, we can agree with the teacher that the child seems to be a bit overly active and has difficulty concentrating. In either case we have said pretty much the same thing. If we should diagnose this condition from a neurological standpoint we have not resolved anything except label the same thing the teacher described. That is the issue. We need to talk about what we can do about it.

Diagnosis in the case of hemispherically related concerns is more a process of observation and development of an understanding of how the child organizes, or fails to organize, and the various aspects of his behavior which seem significant. We need to know about his temperament and personality, about his reading and writing skills (how he attempts them), about his preferences and dislikes, his special interests, something of his early childhood development, how he organizes to solve problems or complete a task, his handedness, when he established dominance, and still many other things. In essence, hemisphericity is not determining which side of the brain he uses, it is rather all those things that the hemispheres are supposed to do and how they are coming together. What we are looking for is a new, at least a more realistic, way of looking at child behavior in order to determine what sorts of teaching strategies are most likely to work and how we will have to treat him in the process. We have to work with a theory in our minds and attempt to compare what we see with what we know about the theory and the child. This will require observations and testing both practical and clinical.

This brings us to an interesting point. One of the greatest problems we see in reviewing school case conference records, and in participating in such reviews, is that the staff does not, or are perhaps not able to, put all of the information together and see the holistic aspects of the child's needs. Diagnostic conferences are almost totally viewed as a "digital" (left brained if you want) process. Diagnosticians have been trained, and by the standardization limits of the tests used, to look at data in a bit by bit viewpoint; consequently they see the trees and not the forest. One of the authors was once told that he did not approach testing as a logical process but rather as an "art." It was perhaps the greatest compliment he had ever received. Diagnosis then presents a good example of why teachers and psychologists are unable to understand the "gestalt" concepts which hemisphericity notions are attempting to communicate.

The typical process of diagnosing learning disabilities is to give a number of individual tests and then to group the data into categories toward identification of the specific problems. These problems are then approached through specific processes of remediation with the hope that somehow it will all finally be put together by the child. Diagnosis *is* an art. It requires that the individual psychologist or team look at the data in a dynamic and holistic process in order to establish overall trends in the child's behavior from which priorities and comprehensive approaches can be initiated. This involves, hemispherically, that the diagnostician use his own left and right hemispheric processes. Through logical processes of observation and testing we obtain the data and then with the synthesis ability of the creative hemisphere we must put together that data into a holistic approach.

Organizing general hemispheric models of potential organization is a somewhat artificial process in that there are many possibilities and because in practice none work out exactly like the model. But it is of value for the diagnostician to have at least some baseline models of potential hemisphericity as an overall theory from which to observe and operate when working with children. A model of hemispheric function must include three major levels of orientation, cerebral dominance, motor-visual dominance, and cerebral efficiency. These three levels need to be discussed briefly before giving some hemispheric models.

CEREBRAL DOMINANCE: Usually, the left hemisphere is dominant in general behavioral organization. This involves a child who is appropriately organized in the socialized mode. This child uses language and language functions to process and evaluate information.

Normally children come, through the sequence of naturalized to socialized development, to utilize dominance in the left hemisphere as their major mode of conscious orientation. The immature child may linger for a longer period of time within naturalized modes as a dominant behavioral style and remain imaginative, creative, disorganized, and impulsive. As the child is developing there are periods where he fluctuates between predominantly naturalized or socialized modes of operation, but eventually he achieves language dominance through left hemispheric development and becomes appropriately socialized.

Some children do not establish good dominance in cerebral function and remain children who are poorly organized and have difficulty with rules, with logical thought, and with general learning skills. Some children finally end with a highly naturalized mode of dominance and become the creative, artistic, athletic, or nonverbally oriented individuals who will continue to have difficulties with organization and social values.

CEREBRAL EFFICIENCY: Due to genetic, environmental, or other causes a child may develop dissonance between the efficiency of the two hemispheres with one or the other becoming much more competent than the other. This results in a significantly higher level of intelligence (competency) in one hemisphere mode than the other.

There is a natural tendency for the left hemisphere to become dominant as was mentioned in the preceding discussion. This usually results in the typical intelligence factor where left hemispheric function displays a higher level of efficiency than the right. The relationship between the two hemispheres determines how the child will process information most efficiently. For example, the child with a verbal I.Q. of 120 is a capable student and though the nonverbal intelligence factor may be lower, he is able to do well in school. There is then a continuous ratio that can be diagnosed through such tests as the WISC-R Intelligence Test. Some examples of such ratios are given here.

A. Verbal I.Q. – 100   Performance (nonverbal) – 100
The theoretical "normal" child.

B. Verbal I.Q. – 110   Performance – 100
The normal child who has experienced good language stimulation.

C. Verbal I.Q. – 120   Performance – 120
The bright child who also exhibits competence in nonverbal intelligence.

D. Verbal I.Q. – 130   Performance – 100
The gifted verbal child with average performance. This child will tend to be highly verbal and have difficulty in areas of nonverbal abilities. He may be an excellent communicator and reader but have problems in school getting things on paper due to poor writing and spatial skills.

E. Verbal I.Q. – 135+   Performance – 135+
The truly all-around gifted child.

These foregoing examples are only general in nature but give an idea of how hemispheric efficiency can affect the child's general performance and mode of orientation in consciousness. The opposite possibility of course also exists.

A. Verbal I.Q. – 100   Performance – 120
The naturalistic tending child who operates from a nonverbal mode of functioning even though he has normal verbal intelligence or efficiency.

B. Verbal I.Q. – 100   Performance – 135+
The so-called Alpha child. This child enjoys creative activities and operates in a highly efficient manner with these functions. His creative intelligence is so high that he avoids verbal learning even though he could accomplish in that area. This child often has difficulty with verbal communication and reading. He enjoys drawing but not writing. He will tend to be impulsive and emotional. This is the creative gifted child.

Other possibilities in hemispheric strategies would include the foregoing areas of competence but coupled with a deficit in the opposite hemisphere.

A. Verbal I.Q. — 100   Performance — 85
   This child has spatial deficits and with only average verbal abilities he may experience many spatially based learning problems.
B. Verbal I.Q. — 85   Performance — 100
   This is the child who has poor language skills and tends to enjoy active learning with a highly sensory-based experience.

These few examples tell us that there are many combinations of hemispheric function, and when there is a significant difference, we have called this cerebral dissonance to suggest that the child's learning and his behavior will be affected by the difference in efficiency between the major hemisphere functions. If genetic factors create the difference, then the child may be highly resistant to stimulation of the deficit or lower hemispheric function and have to be taught differently. These differences can be caused by environment, deprivation, or enhancement, and they also usually affect or are caused by emotional factors.

If hemispheric dominance or efficiency were the end of the matter all would be far simpler. Unfortunately, the additional concern of motor and visual dominance must also be considered and adds a great deal of influence to the processing of information. Left– and right–handedness also play a strong role and complicate the diagnosis of the child's needs. There are many possible motoric strategies that a child may use in relation to the cerebral dominance factors.

The normal child utilizes a left hemispheric cerebral dominance with right hand and eye dominance. (See Figure 2-A.) The dominant hemisphere in cerebral function is usually also the most efficient hemisphere and it is normally the hemisphere that determines hand dominance. The left hemispheric child is usually right-handed and the right hemispheric child is usually left-handed. But alas, it is not that simple. Before attacking that problem a brief review of the effects of handedness on learning should be presented.

Ontogenetic development dictates that learning to control the parts of the body in motor function proceeds from the head to the toes and from the middle of the body out to the extremities. This is a simple fact of physiology we have all known for a long time. But what affect does this have on cerebral orientation and organization? Lots! The process of developing motor control from the middle of the body out also establishes, in the brain, an orientation of spatial-directional preference. In that the right hand develops from the middle out to the right (left to right) this also organizes a neuro pattern of working most easily from left to right and hence the pattern of right-handed children writing and working from left to right. But the left-handed child also develops from the middle out and establishes a pattern of organization that is mostly natural from the right to the left. When the left-handed child writes from the right to the left or reverses letters he is not writing backwards, he is writing forwards for the left–handed pattern of neuro organization. He has to learn to write "backwards" in order to write like a right-handed child does.

Since the dominant hand is usually associated with the dominant hemisphere, hand dominance is usually an indication of cerebral dominance, but it may not be. The left-handed child usually is dominant in right hemispheric motor function but he may or may not be dominant in right hemispheric cerebral function. To further complicate things, the right-handed child is usually left hemispheric dominant in cerebral function, but many children are not! Now that creates a great deal of confusion for the bit-by-bit diagnostician who is himself usually well organized.

It is the relationship between cerebral dominance and motor dominance that often creates many of the directional, spatial, and fine motor problems of children, not to mention many difficulties in sequence and time. We call this relationship the cerebral-motor dominance factor. This factor is one that many teachers and psychologists have difficulty understanding, because it does create a bit of confusion when one tries to remember the various aspects of dominance that are involved. But this particular aspect of hemisphericity is the key to a great many learning problems of children.

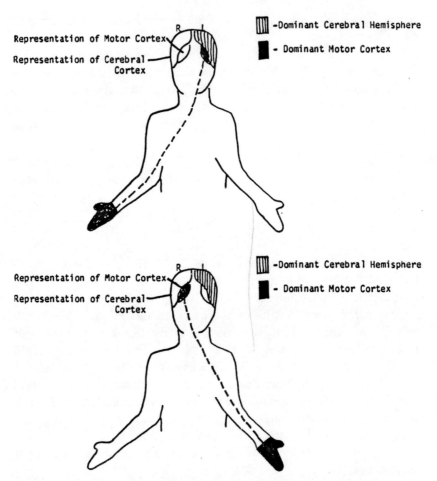

Figure 2-A. Typical right-handed child. Characteristics: Right handed, left cerebral dominant. The typical right-handed child is dominant in the language hemisphere. This is the expected neurological arrangement where the hand is controlled by the same side hemisphere as that in which language is usually located. This child is able to perform motor functions "naturally" from left to right and has normal orientation to language-based concepts of thought and general orientation.

Figure 2-B. Typical left-handed child. Left handed, left cerebral dominant. The typical left-handed child, though dominant in the right motor area resulting in left handedness, is still dominant in left hemispheric language, and therefore differs from the typical right-handed child only in the right motor dominance resulting in left handedness. The left-handed child is language oriented and is able to reason through the reversal needed to work left-to-right even though the tendency to work right-to-left is dictated by the right hemispheric dominance. This child, being language oriented is able to organize his world appropriately and learn in a typical school environment.

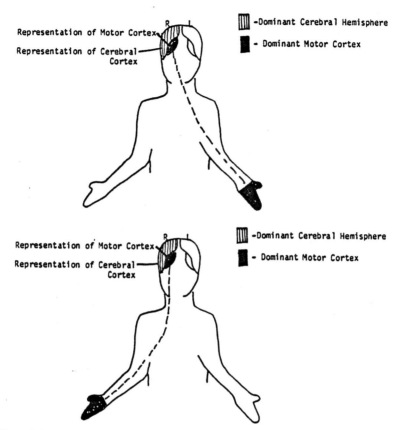

Representation of Motor Cortex
Representation of Cerebral Cortex

[||||] -Dominant Cerebral Hemisphere
[■] - Dominant Motor Cortex

Representation of Motor Cortex
Representation of Cerebral Cortex

[||||] -Dominant Cerebral Hemisphere
[■] - Dominant Motor Cortex

Figure 2-C. The totally left-handed child. Characteristics: This is a child who is not only right motoric dominant resulting in left-handedness, but he is also right cerebrally dominant. In such a child language function is often found in both left and right hemispheres, but the predominant mental orientation is naturalistic and nonverbal. These children tend to be very creative, enjoy art and music, tend to like active games such as sports, and may exhibit much emotionality.

The totally left-handed child may represent a genetic difference and this may account for his often extreme resistance both to changing hands and to learning adequate language-based functions. This child has difficulty learning left-right organizations and learning to adapt to the structure of a classroom.

Figure 2-D. The naturalistic right-handed child. Characteristics: Right handed but total right hemispheric dominance.

The naturalistic child is right handed but internal organization is exactly the same as the totally left-handed child. Further, this child is also poorly organized in language and displays a significantly higher nonverbal, right hemispheric competency, making him a very emotional, creative, impulsive, and active child.

This child has tremendous problems in spatial motor organization and in language skills. While the totally left-handed child can be a problem for himself and the teacher, the naturalistic child is even more difficult.

The right hemisphere tends to organize information either nondirectionally, holistically, or from a right to left pattern as with the left-handed child. The left hemisphere tends to organize information in a left-to-right pattern. Those are the essential facts that underpin the cerebral-motor dominance factor. If that is kept in mind the problem is less difficult. Now let's look at some of the problems that can become active when a child has either mixed cerebral and hand dominance or motor and visual dominance, or both.

Let us look at the four basic patterns of cerebral-motor organization that we most often see in children and note the various problems that certain patterns create for children.

In Figure 2-A we saw the basic "model" of cerebral-motor organization. This is the child as children are "supposed" to be, according to the world we live in. Here the child is right-handed and utilizes the left hemisphere motor area to control the right hand along with demonstrating left hemispheric motoric strategies that make "sense" because they are organized in the same pattern as is his basic neurological structure. Learning letters, organizing time, sequential thought organization, and reading will all move from left to right in the same manner as his basic "natural" tendencies.

In Figure 2-B we see the typical left-handed child. This child utilizes right hemispheric motor dominance and his left hand. However, this child is left hemispheric dominant in general cerebral organization like the typical right-handed child and therefore the left-handed orientation is primarily limited to motor function.

Left-handed children have been a problem for the culture throughout time. There has been a long history in education and within families to attempt to prevent children from using their left hands and we have long attempted to "force" left-handed children to switch before beginning school. We continue to see a surprising number of children whose parents admit that they forced the child to use his right hand.

In the past left-handed children were often seen as "backward" and possessors of many unusual behaviors and/or personality traits. In our work with left-handed children we have observed a great range of behavioral and learning patterns which, without some organizing theory, seemed confusing and without any consistency from child to child. We are going to present here two sorts of left-handed children who do consistently display specific behavioral traits and then a final pattern of a right-handed child who also is in reality a left-handed child.

There are two levels of left-handedness. The first level is represented by Figure 2-B. While the child is left-handed, he exhibits typical left hemispheric mental organization patterns. In essence, the language appears dominant and the child experiences no particular difficulty with language or speech but has some problems in early school experience with motor organization, producing reversed letters, reading some words and letters backwards, and some difficulty in learning time or temporally related skills. Generally though, these children are able to work out their difficulties with practice and patience.

In Figure 2-C we see another left-handed child, but he represents another type and perhaps should truly be called a natural left-handed child. The child in Figure 2-C is one of not only right motor dominance but also right hemispheric dominant.

The Figure 2-C child has higher efficiency and competence in right hemispheric function and, although there may be adequate language function, the right hemisphere mode of organization is dominant. This is quite a different matter than the left-handed child (Figure 2-B) who is motorically left-handed but still has left cerebral dominance. The Figure 2-B child still has cerebral organization which is appropriate to the left to right organization in cognitive or mental function. But the Figure 2-C child is a truly different child in that he is predominantly organized around spatial-creative thought patterns. Though he may recognize that he writes letters backwards or reverses other motor responses, he has difficulty understanding why he should change. Most often the child will simply avoid all sequential and language-based activities. He will have trouble maintaining attention since he does not utilize the left hemispheric function to organize his behavior. This child exhibits all of the naturalistic thought and behavioral patterns as outlined in Figure 2-C. This sort of child has great difficulty in school and only through persistence of teachers and parents is he able to complete his schoolwork at all. This group of conditions is more difficult to deal with than the Figure 2-B conditions where only motor dominance is left. But this would be expected for these children are truly different in the basis used for mental organization. They tend to view the world with a perceptual– and activity-based attitude seeking novelty, musical, athletic, artistic, or activity based interests. They have great difficulty in phonetics due to their inability to sequence sounds and information easily. It would appear that Figure 2-C children have a stronger dose of genetic tendency than the Figure 2-B children, and therefore they are more resistive to enculturation toward changing hands or attending to language-based function.

We have been struck by this basic difference in many left-handed children: some are primarily motoric left-handers but language based, while others are totally right hemispheric in both motor and in general cerebral organization. Our assumption, that Figure 2-C left-handedness is more deeply rooted in the genetic structure is, of course, only speculation. But the basis for the difference is perhaps less important to educators and psychologists than the fact that these two types do exist. Both can benefit from early assistance in developing more skilled left to right function. However, the Figure 2-C left-handed child is very resistive to attempts to make him more organized and to learn the skills required to write and read. The difference in the two children can usually be observed behaviorally, but administration of the WISC-R Intelligence Test, and an analysis of fine motor skills and reading style, will often verify the difference in the two children.

The Figure 2-C children frequently must begin different approaches to reading and general schoolwork. Often they do better initially with a whole-word language experience approach, because they do have good fantasy and visual imagery and can make up stories easily. This encourages them to use and develop language function and, at the same time, allows them more motivation because of the attention and recognition they receive. The stories are then broken into whole word approaches that the child can more easily handle with the gestalt tendencies than the bit by bit phonetic approach. After a year or so these children can then be moved into phonetics and appear to do well. All of this, along with the specific motor exercises and activities, eventually moves them from a primarily right hemispheric orientation to at least a more acceptable language-based approach to their environment. Yet, these children remain very creative and impulsive, artistic or musical, and often exhibit much emotionality to their environment. The behavioral management of these children is difficult for parents and teachers, and many adults finally give up and try to threaten or force them into the conventional learning and behavioral mode. It usually does not work. Helping these children requires much support, love, and structure in following through with practice and effort.

The Figure 2-C left-handed child has a severe reaction to parents or teachers who attempt to force him to use his right hand. Unlike the Figure 2-B left-handed child who can often make the switch with only minimal negative consequences, the Figure 2-C child simply will not do so and will offer such resistance that adults usually give up.

These two types of left-handed children both display a somewhat distinct movement from the typical right-handed child to a greater and greater developmental difference. But there is one more type, and as you might guess, the most severe difference of the four is exhibited with this child. The Figure 2-D child is the Figure 2-C child who, for whatever reason, genetic or environmental, has in fact learned to use the right hand. The significant problem, though, is that this child is a right motor and cerebral hemispheric child who controls the right hand through ipsilateral control, that is, he controls the right hand with the right motor hemisphere. This is the child who was the subject of our book on Alpha children, because this is a frequently encountered child, and he presents a most difficult diagnostic problem for psychologists who do not have some working knowledge of hemisphericity.

On the WISC-R Intelligence Test, which gives both a verbal and nonverbal readout, the Figure 2-D child often displays a much higher nonverbal (right hemispheric) level of competency than in verbal abilities. Again, it is not so important that we can prove that the high nonverbal intellectual score truly even represents right hemispheric function, though this is somewhat well established, but rather that the child does do much better on spatial

tasks than on verbal tasks. For example, the following characteristics are often common in the Figure 2-D child.

1. Significantly higher spatial than verbal intelligence (at least
   15 points but usually more than 20).
2. Tends to have difficulty in form drawing but often is quite
   good in freehand drawings. These, even though accuracy
   may not be good, display a high degree of conceptualiza-
   tion in imagery. This means that the drawings show much
   elaboration, such as details, movement, costumes, and
   action or emotion.
3. Tends to approach words through a whole word and guess
   technique and makes many whole word substitutions.
4. Is very sensitive and tends to be emotional, moving from
   highs to lows quickly. He is impulsive and demanding of
   peers.
5. He may reverse letters or write letters out of sequence, and
   has trouble learning the time and sequence of days and
   months.
6. He has a good sense of humor and often enjoys active and
   loud play.
7. He often tries to dominate or direct peers.
8. He has a rich imagination and ability to fantasize.
9. He enjoys music, drama, and art activities.
10. He loves to pretend, make funny noises, and play with
    animals.

These are but a few of the characteristics that these children
exhibit. There are others and many are specific to areas of skill
and learning difficulties. Many of the children exhibit some, and
others all, of these characteristics. These are very predictable
when we consider the general functions of right hemispheric organization. These can be very loving and affectionate children, because like right hemispheric function suggests, they rely on touch
and affection for communication with those they like.

These four types of children illustrate an important point in
the diagnosis of hemisphericity and the issue cannot be discussed
too much. Much of the present literature on diagnosis of hemispheric difference involves two directions of emphasis; in education, how to increase the right hemispheric or supposed deficit

many children suffer in this sort of learning, and, in psychometrics, how to pinpoint hemispheric differences in testing, i.e. the WISC-R, which suggest a deficit in one or the other hemispheric function. Both of these approaches have value in working with children, but both still miss the point. Analysis and understanding of hemispheric organization in a specific case is not a major goal but rather adding the hemispheric theory and data to a range of additional information about the child to better understand his overall educational and developmental needs.

As we have suggested, hemispheric differences also carry with them probable differences in perceptual motor organization, sequential thought, temporal organization, and, as we will see, personality as well. Hemispheric theory then provides a more encompassing point of reference upon which the general development and behavior of the child can be understood. If application of hemispheric theory seems to be inaccurate, or, even worse, incorrect in a specific case; then the diagnostician has poorly understood the overall intent and nature of the theory and is applying it, as we fear, as a new unified theory of human behavior. It is not a unified theory but rather a part of the overall neurological development of the child.

Psychometrists are referred to an excellent publication concerning the specific analysis of hemisphericity in the use of the WISC-R Intelligence Test called *Intelligent Testing with the WISC-R*, by Alan Kaufman, published by Wiley and Sons. For the psychometrist that publication gives a valuable viewpoint concerning how to use the WISC-R within the context of overall analysis of hemispheric techniques. Specific analysis of subtests is well outlined. But for our purposes here we will talk in more general terms, since our intent is to assist the teacher and psychologist in the overall understanding of the theory within the educational setting. It is important though to point out that materials are available to the psychometrist in specific subtest data.

As will be seen in the case studies the critical aspects of diagnosis of hemispheric factors are those contained within a range of instruments and techniques extending beyond the typical psychometric assessment. This point is well made in Kaufman's book, although that publication does focus primarily on the WISC-R itself. In this book we intend to focus, though we will include aspects of the WISC-R, on the broader range of approaches both formal and informal in making an analysis of the child's needs.

The process we have used, while including the WISC-R and other formal tests, when looking at the development of children, includes a range of information which is listed here. This information is obtained through a variety of approaches, and often duplicate tests will be used to look at a specific factor from several modes of behavior.

1. Family history, including peculiarities of the parents or relatives in developmental and learning behaviors.
2. Early development in motor-perceptual function.
3. Fine and gross motor abilities and skills.
4. Creative abilities in both formal and informal drawing activities.
5. Verbal and spatial intelligence, i.e. WISC-R.
6. Spatial-directional orientation and competency.
7. Verbal expression and language fluency.
8. Flexibility in approach to task analysis and completion in relation to the nature of the task.
9. General personality style and interpersonal modes.
10. General moral development and value orientations.
11. Intra-family interaction and role.

Each of these areas can shed significant light on a child's needs or his problem. In each area one could spend hours of time accumulating data and attempting to analyze it. In our work we attempt to scan these areas looking for both overall competencies and deficits and relationships to the child's current functioning and making predictions concerning potentialities in the child's development. These areas are screened in a general way and specific areas in which difficulties are noted are given more attention. From the overall screening, assumptions are made concerning the child's needs and specific programming recommendations are made. Following the overall evaluation the teacher then proceeds to work on the assumption given, as do the parents, with a continuous process of reassessment and reorganization of the child's programming. The process then includes first an overall global process in which the general picture can be established. Following that, specifics are developed. Too often a diagnostic approach includes administration of many hours of testing and specific data collection after which everyone is overwhelmed by the amount of data. We find that too much specific data is accumulated in a "standardized" diagnostic process, which cannot or should not be used. We find that the more holistic assessment with general checking of many areas without in-depth testing often eliminates many useless hours of simply giving every test in the book, because that is what the psychometrist usually does. Again, it is the digital analysis versus the analog analysis, concrete first, and then abstract, and back to concrete. Look at what is observable, change it into data if needed, and then go back to the observable.

Within the area of making an analysis of hemispheric differences, in cerebral dominance, and cerebral dissonance (when one hemisphere is significantly more competent than the other) there are many strategies that can be used. The following strategies are somewhat general but give a number of observable factors which can be of assistance to the teacher and psychologist who are making such an analysis. This is not an exhaustive list nor is it all that the authors use but it will provide a basic introduction to the concept and then in the case studies additional factors will be discussed.

We must remind the reader that our interest in this book is primarily with the naturalistic child and not with the highly socialized child. Most of our discussions will center about understanding and identifying the highly naturalistic child. However, problems do exist with the child who is overly socialized and who demonstrates excellent and high left hemispheric function. Often that is the child that much of the literature is presently focusing on. The concept of generally improving the creative and naturalistic abilities of children with depressed function in this area is one of the major directions in the area of left-right brain theory and a proliferation of literature is beginning to flood the market in this orientation. We do not need to add to the material. Conversely, the child who is already creative and highly naturalistic without adequate language function is the child for whom this book is written. We do not take issue with the general trend to improve naturalistic function, quite the contrary, it is an important and needed development in education because it involves critical human behavior. Yet, there are significant numbers of what we called Alpha children, and in the present glut of interest in developing creative abilities, these children, who already have too much of a good thing, are suffering with the general educational interest missing them altogether. The following factors then are pointed to discovering these children and understanding how to help them.

The following checklist, used for observation in the classroom, is a general, though imperfect, means of looking at the functions within verbal and creative behavioral areas. Scoring is less important than the process of looking at the general behaviors of the child to see if there is a difference in the two major realms of behavior. Following the completion of this general survey the teacher can then solicit the aid of the psychometrist in doing more detailed and complete analysis.

Hemispheric Observation Guide

Factor Socialized Mode

A. Verbal expressive   1 2 3 4
    1. Displays appropriate vocabulary for age.   _ _ _ _
    2. Speaks with good syntax and language structure. _ _ _ _
    3. Answers specific questions adequately.   _ _ _ _
    4. Describes personal thoughts in proper sequence. _ _ _ _
    5. Asks questions in order to obtain information. _ _ _ _
B. Logical
    1. Shows objectivity in attitude toward others.   _ _ _ _
    2. Evaluates situation and personal behavior.   _ _ _ _
    3. Recognizes consequences of personal behavior.   _ _ _ _
    4. Selects appropriate goals and personal behavior. _ _ _ _
    5. Understands reasons for rules.   _ _ _ _
C. Orderly and sequential
    1. Recalls a series of directions.   _ _ _ _
    2. Follows a series of directions.   _ _ _ _
    3. Displays appropriate personal organization.   _ _ _ _
    4. Displays sequential pattern of thought.   _ _ _ _
    5. Predicts outcomes of behavior.   _ _ _ _

D. Time orientation   1 2 3 4
    1. Knows sequence of days, weeks, months, or time of day.   _ _ _ _
    2. Understands and uses numbers appropriate for age.   _ _ _ _
    3. Aware of and adheres to time-related activities.   _ _ _ _
    4. Paces personal activities to time limits.   _ _ _ _
    5. Uses time to organize self.   _ _ _ _

E. Socialized values
    1. Recognizes and uses appropriate social behaviors. _ _ _ _
    2. Understands situational rules of right and wrong. _ _ _ _
    3. Displays appropriate remorse or guilt for behavior.   _ _ _ _
    4. Strives for social acceptance.   _ _ _ _
    5. Has socially appropriate and acceptable goals.   _ _ _ _

F. Aggressive and assertive
    1. Is personally assertive with others.   _ _ _ _
    2. Has a desire to compete.   _ _ _ _
    3. Concerned about fair play and cooperative.   _ _ _ _
    4. Appears to want rules in games and work.   _ _ _ _
    5. Shows personal motivation to achieve.   _ _ _ _

G. Abstract thought
    1. Can discuss relationships in abstract terms.   _ _ _ _
    2. Can apply rules to abstract situations.   _ _ _ _
    3. Enjoys mathematical games and tasks.   _ _ _ _
    4. Can discuss remote relationships.   _ _ _ _
    5. Displays logical problem-solving ability.   _ _ _ _

H. Vertical thought — structured
    1. Can apply rules to problems in math.   _ _ _ _
    2. Can predict outcomes in familiar situations.   _ _ _ _
    3. Displays deductive ability.   _ _ _ _
    4. Is able to classify and categorize information.   _ _ _ _
    5. Displays understanding of social behavior consequences.   _ _ _ _

I. Objective
    1. Can use criteria to evaluate situations or information.   _ _ _ _
    2. Learns and uses social rules.   _ _ _ _

	1	2	3	4

3. Displays a lack of bias in appropriate situations.   _ _ _ _
4. Can remove self from situation and evaluation.   _ _ _ _
5. Can listen and accept viewpoints of others.   _ _ _ _

J. Conventional motor organization
  1. Organizes work appropriately from left to right.   _ _ _ _
  2. Uses right-handed mode of writing.   _ _ _ _
  3. Able to read or sequence left to right without
     difficulty.   _ _ _
  4. Organizes work well on paper with proper spacing
     and size.   _ _ _ _
  5. Has good balance and coordination.   _ _ _ _

Factor Naturalized Mode

A. Motorically expressive
  1. Enjoys physical activities and games.   _ _ _ _
  2. Likes to draw, paint, build, and make things.   _ _ _ _
  3. Relates to others physically; touching; hitting.   _ _ _ _
  4. Talks with many gestures and physical
     movements.   _ _ _ _
  5. Displays general restlessness during verbal or
     highly structured situations.   _ _ _ _

B. Intuitive
  1. Exhibits high sensitivity to the feelings of others.   _ _ _ _
  2. Displays frequent mood changes, appears
     introspective, daydreams, and gains insight about
     others.   _ _ _ _
  3. Sees the practical basis of a problem.   _ _ _ _
  4. Highly responsive to music and situational mood.   _ _ _ _
  5. Highly aware of sensory information in the
     environment (tastes, smells, color, etc).   _ _ _ _

C. Holistic and gestalt
  1. Sees a higher purpose or general goals but may
     miss specific goals or sequence of behavior.   _ _ _ _
  2. Attempts to understand complex situations in a
     general way without regard for details.   _ _ _ _
  3. Perceives whole words, phrases, and sentences.   _ _ _ _
  4. Has general feeling about pictures or objects but
     can remember few details.   _ _ _ _

1 2 3 4

    5. Remembers visual aspect of people and objects
       but can remember few details.   _ _ _ _

D. Spatial orientation
    1. Highly sophisticated visual memory; knows and
       describes past events but cannot remember dates,
       time, or names.   _ _ _ _
    2. Has excellent movement capacity in activities.   _ _ _ _
    3. Orients to either right or left without defined
       preferences or outside supervision.   _ _ _ _
    4. Good directional orientation but good memory
       for physical characteristics of past locations.   _ _ _ _
    5. Enjoys open spaces and lack of crowding.   _ _ _ _

E. Naturalistic values
    1. Uses situational values rather than cultural norms._ _ _ _
    2. Considers experiences of value if they are
       self-stimulating.   _ _ _ _
    3. Has a need for immediate gratification.   _ _ _ _
    4. Tends to see self as important and as the center of
       all things. Feels a oneness with all.   _ _ _ _
    5. Displays shifting friendships, on-off depending on
       personal moods at the time.   _ _ _ _

F. Submissive and accepting
    1. Tends to be accepting of others without personal
       commitment to them, autonomous.   _ _ _ _
    2. Tends to accept aggression without a need to
       counter.   _ _ _ _
    3. Submits to compromise rather than conflict.   _ _ _ _
    4. Changes goals if extensive blocking occurs.   _ _ _ _
    5. Becomes aggressive when others try to direct him
       but will submit if he simply has to stop activity. _ _ _ _

G. Concrete thought
    1. Displays apparent high degree of "common
       sense."   _ _ _ _
    2. Tends to state things as they are.   _ _ _ _
    3. Tends to need sensory input with information.   _ _ _ _
    4. Socially astute.   _ _ _ _
    5. Has difficulty seeing remote relationships.   _ _ _ _

H. Lateral thought — creative   1 2 3 4
    1. Tends to be imaginative and fantasy oriented.   _ _ _ _
    2. Develops unusual responses and solutions.   _ _ _ _
    3. Tends to develop a variety of thoughts surrounding
       one stimulus.   _ _ _ _
    4. Tends to automatically elaborate on ideas.   _ _ _ _
    5. Can visualize and create unusual "things."   _ _ _ _
I. Subjective
    1. Relates goals to self.   _ _ _ _
    2. Evaluates others on the basis of personal beliefs.   _ _ _ _
    3. Embues objectives and others with personal
       characteristics.   _ _ _ _
    4. Often responds in a highly emotional way to
       situations of stress or conflict.   _ _ _ _
    5. Determined to believe personal values and
       constructs.   _ _ _ _
J. Mixed and Unconventional motor organization
    1. Has a tendency to reverse letters or the order of
       letters.   _ _ _ _
    2. Has a tendency to use a different hand for various
       tasks.   _ _ _ _
    3. Displays visual-motor difficulty in fine motor
       tasks that are educationally structured but not in
       personal activity.   _ _ _ _
    4. Has a tendency to reverse spoken words in syntax
       or in writing.   _ _ _ _
    5. Good organization skills in written work and in
       general behavior. (1)   _ _ _ _

One of the most important areas of investigation is that of seeking information about the family history of both mother and father concerning their own general mode of organization and any significant difficulties they may have experienced. Are the parents both left-handed? Are there many left-handed people on one side of the family or the other? Did either parent have significant difficulties early in school, in reading or writing? Is there a history of dyslexia in the family or were there special areas of academic development that either parent found difficult? Is either of the parents a highly naturalistic individual? In essence we are searching to see if either parent demonstrated as a child or now demonstrates behavior which would suggest genetic and family-based differences. The following questions, within this context, are usually asked of the parents.

Parent Questionnaire

1. What is the incidence of left-handedness within the immediate family and relatives?
2. Did either parent develop language or learn to talk late?
3. Did the child talk late? What were the characteristics of the early language of the child?
4. Did the child show an early interest in creative activities such as imagination, drawing, building, animals, or gross motor activities?
5. At what age did the child take his first steps, speak his first words, and were there unusual accomplishments in this area?
6. Describe the masculine and feminine nature of the child's early behavior.
7. Does the child go to sleep easily or does he attempt to stay up late?
8. Does the child enjoy television and fantasy material?
9. Is the child a science fiction buff?
10. Did the child have difficulty selecting a dominant hand? At what age did he do so?
11. Does he enjoy playmates and does he get along with other children?
12. Does he tend to dominate others in play?
13. Does he tend to become angry when others do not do what he wants to do?
14. Is he emotional? Does he tend to get frustrated or angry easily and then get over it quickly?
15. Does he have trouble remembering directions given to him at school or at home?
16. Does he sometimes forget what he was planning to do due to a distraction?
17. Is he highly affectionate?
18. Does he like animals but tend to forget to take care of them?

19. Does he daydream a lot?
20. Does he make up stories or enjoy telling fantastic and imaginative stories?

The highly naturalistic child tends to display all or many of the above characteristics. We find that highly creative and naturalistic children tend to engage in many of these behaviors, and while some are characteristic of all children at times, the more extensively the child engages in these behaviors to the exclusion of opposite behaviors the more likely it is we are seeing a child who is organized within naturalistic function.

One of the most striking factors in the parent interview concerning these factors is that often the father describes his own childhood as being very much like that of the child.

EARLY PERCEPTUAL MOTOR DEVELOPMENT

The highly naturalistic child, as described by the four types in the preceding discussion, often experiences directional, spatial, and specific motoric difficulties. As the child is given various tests, specific factors are observed that point to these difficulties. Obviously, often these characteristics will be observed in a number of specific behaviors and the following activities provide excellent opportunities to observe such difficulties.

1. The child is asked to touch his left ear with his right hand. Often the child will have difficulty with this. Although he may eventually figure out the movement, there is often a significant pause as the child moves first one hand and then the other.
2. The use of the preferred hand is observed throughout all motoric activities.
3. The child is asked to stand on one foot with his eyes open and closed to determine his ability to balance using visual feedback and kinesthetic feedback. This demonstrates his basic balance and kinesthetic efficiency.
4. The child is asked to draw a person. Factors to observe during this activity are:
   a. Does he draw from the bottom up? This is often an indicator of spatial difficulty and yet some children will do

this because they feel more comfortable in working from the bottom up just as they feel more comfortable working from right to left.

b. Does the child draw a stick person? Often naturalistic children will do this because they don't like to draw people or because they have little interest in doing something for someone else. Naturalistic children often enjoy drawing things like space vehicles or cars which fit more into their general interests.

c. Does the child elaborate the drawing including other things in the picture, showing movement and/or expression, or some unique characteristic? In general, brighter and more creative children do this, of course.

d. Some naturalistic children take great pains in this sort of drawing and attempt to make a realistic and capable drawing because they enjoy art.

e. Often we also ask a child to draw and color any picture he wants in order to see the difference between doing a structured task and one that he may enjoy more. Often the difference is startling and we learn much more from the free choice drawing than the formal Draw-A-Person Test. But we ask the child to do both.

Formal drawing tests include the Berry Developmental Test, and the Bender Gestalt. In asking children to draw forms we almost always ask them to do so freehand and with the instructions that there will be several drawings. On the Berry they copy a drawing within a box and are limited. This often misses some of the following critical points or organization skills; therefore, even with the Berry, we ask them to simply do the drawings on a piece of plain white paper. The following points are observed as they draw.

a. Is the *size appropriate* or are the drawings made larger than the models, suggesting a more expansive style or a lack of fine motor control?

b. Some children with poor motoric skills will *make the drawings larger and larger* and have more difficulty as they continue with the task, indicating a lack of endurance and overall fine motor skill.

c. Children with directional and fine motor difficulties will often have many *problems with the angles* and end up putting "tails" on the diamonds or squares indicating a lack of good spatial and motor organization. We often have the child practice for a moment if this happens to see if cueing and assistance improve the effort. This often is one sign that assures us that the child is having difficulties in maturation rather than actual neurological problems. The naturalistic child will often show immediate improvement while the child with neurological problems will continue to experience problems.

d. Does the child *place the forms in a left to right order* and in a *fairly organized* pattern? Naturalistic children often focus on each drawing and place the forms in a random pattern with little regard for left to right placement and overall organization. Again, children with learning disabilities will do this because they have difficulties with spatial organization. The naturalistic child can organize the pattern but simply does not attend to overall structure.

e. Does the child place the drawings in a *vertical pattern*? This often indicates an avoidance of the left-to-right organization and is not uncommon with the naturalistic child. It is not that he cannot organize but rather that he simply avoids doing so in favor of concentrating on the forms themselves.

The reader should be reminded time and again throughout these discussions that we are pointing the general discussion toward both teachers and psychometrists or psychologists and therefore there will often be too little depth for psychologists. Our intent is to assist the teacher in gaining knowledge about *general* concepts of testing so that the teacher and the psychologist can work together from at least common understandings concerning diagnostic procedures. Many of the tests and procedures can be done by the teacher in the classroom while others will have to be done by psychologists. The psychologist will be able to extend the analysis far beyond much of the discussion here, yet this information should help the psychologist and teacher to reach a common ground upon which to make an analysis. The teacher, after all, will be the one who must provide the assistance, and it is important for him or her to have at least some grasp of both the things he or she can do and those that will be done by the psychologist. For example, the teacher can accomplish some general drawing analysis but such tests as the Bender Gestalt would have to be administered by the psychometrist.

Another point that should be continuously clarified is that many of the characteristics of the naturalistic child who is highly right hemispheric will be similar to those of the immature child in verbal and spatial organization. In that respect then any child, naturalistic or immature, will respond to the same techniques of remediation assistance. The focus of our analysis is that of the naturalistic child, but in many cases immature children will suffer from the same problems as the naturalistic child. Our task in both cases is to improve the efficiency of naturalistic functions while also improving the verbal skills. Again, this is counter to much of the prevailing interest in right hemispheric functions, where the popular concept is to improve the naturalistic function of children who generally have adequate verbal skills.

WISC-R Intelligence Test

Verbal and spatial intelligence or efficiency: The WISC-R Intelligence Test is divided into verbal and spatial tests and yields I.Q. scores for each major area. Both the verbal and spatial areas include six subtests. A general summary of these subtests is presented here.

In our work we utilize the verbal and spatial portions as representative of the major areas of hemispheric functions. The cerebral dissonance syndrome cited in our earlier work suggested that significant differences in the functioning of the two hemispheres could be roughly interpreted as differences in hemispheric capability or, as we termed it, cerebral dissonance. Our assumption was that a significant difference of 15 points or more indicated that the child would have a tendency to favor management of sensory information from the most efficient hemisphere. We still hold to that concept and use it as a *general* measure. However, merely because there is such a difference in itself is not used as

A Description of the WISC-R Subtests

Subtest	Description of a Typical Task	Functions tested	Influencing factors
Verbal Scale			
Information	"What is a play?"	Long-term memory, association and organization of experience	Cultural environment, interests
Comprehension	"Why do we wash clothes?"	Reasoning with abstraction; organization of knowledge; concept formation	Cultural opportunities; response to reality situations
Arithmetic	"How many inches are there in ½ foot?"	Retention of arithmetic processes; attention span	Opportunity to acquire the fundamental arithmetic processes
Vocabulary	"What does mammal mean?"	Language development; concept formation	Cultural opportunities
Digit Span	Repeat digits forward and backwards	Immediate recall; auditory imagery; visual imagery at times	Attention span
Similarities	"In what way is a bicycle like a car?"	Analysis of relationships; verbal concept formation	Cultural opportunities
Performance Scale			
Picture Arrangement	Arrangement of related pictures to form a cartoon-like story	Visual perception of relationships; synthesis of nonverbal material	A minimum of cultural opportunities; visual acuity
Picture Completion	Name the important missing part in each of a series of pictures	Visual perception; visual imagery	Environmental experience; visual acuity at times
Object Assembly	A puzzle task in which the child takes a familiar pattern and puts it together to form a meaningful whole (duck, cow)	Visual perception: synthesis, visual-motor integration	Rate and perception of motor acuity
Block Design	Construction of designs with colored blocks	Perception of form; visual perception and analysis, visual motor integration	Rate of motor activity; minimum of color vision
Coding	Pairing symbols with numbers according to a sample	Immediate recall; visual-motor integration; visual imagery	Rate of motor activity
Mazes	Finding a pathway through a paper maze pattern	Ability to plan ahead; freedom from distraction	Rate and precision of motor activity; anxiety

the sole criterion. Rather, the difference along with the range of information and behavioral observations is used. There are several reasons for this and some are strictly clinical in the validity of stating that the two sections of the WISC-R actually distinctly measure hemispheric difference. They do not. For example, picture completion and block design require much verbal explanation, and the picture completion requires sequential ability, which is usually assigned to verbal abilities. Thus, there is, in the usual method of testing, much verbal contamination of the spatial tests rendering them less than accurate as a measure of only naturalistic or spatial intelligence. In essence, clinically, the concept that each major section measures only verbal or spatial intelligence respectfully is not accurate. Yet, when used in conjunction with a number of other indicators as outlined here, we find that the evaluator can use the difference in spatial and verbal intelligence as a major indicator. We again refer the psychologist to Kaufman's book concerning the clinical application of the WISC-R results in this area. For the teacher, however, we encourage using the difference as a general indicator as we will do throughout our examples of case studies. When the differences increase to levels exceeding perhaps 20 or more points, it is our experience that we are in fact seeing a fairly valid indicator of cerebral difference. Conversely, we have observed many children who demonstrate less than a five-point difference who, on all other indicators, demonstrated a significant right hemispheric or naturalistic orientation. In areas of minor differences then the additional indicators become more important and in the case of significant difference such indicators may be less important.

Use of the WISC-R subtest scores will be demonstrated in more detail in the actual discussion of case studies. Avoiding for a moment the specifics, there are a number of indicators that we have found very important not in the specific subtest scores but rather in the administration and task activity of the child while taking the test. The following factors are those that we have found important as indicators of a highly right hemispheric child during the administration of the WISC-R.

The Naturalistic Child's Performance

a. Naturalistic children often have difficulty with the information subtest. This subtest involves recall of specific verbal information. In our experience children who have high spatial capacities often have difficulty in specific verbal recall. This is due to the spatial confusion these children often exhibit. Specific recall of verbal information is accomplished through a sort of "mental directional" search for information. When there is spatial confusion the child has difficulty recalling specific verbal information, almost as if his filing system is out of order due to confusion. This is important not so much in the score a child received but in the difficulty the child had recalling the information.

b. Many naturalistic children are somewhat dependent upon perceptual information and often have difficulty seeing abstract relationships, even though they are capable of doing so. For example, in similarities if we ask a child how a carrot and a beet are alike they respond with such things as, "They grow in the ground, you eat them both," or "They both have leaves." These are perceptual characteristics. The best answer is the abstract response that they are both vegetables. If the child is told that they are both vegetables he may continue to give perceptual characteristics on the following items, but with some cueing will immediately come up with the appropriate abstraction. The cueing can be done after the subtest is scored and the test completed. The additional effort gives the examiner the information that the child may tend to "think" preferably in perceptual terms, while he is capable of abstraction. Again, clinically there may be a number of reasons for this but when reinforced by many other indicators this can help identify the naturalistic thinker.

c. The naturalistic child is very dependent upon concrete sensory information and it is not surprising that he is often the last child to give up the use of fingers in counting and in general math. Often on the WISC this child will utilize his fingers in nearly all problems in order to obtain concrete feedback in counting.

d. In vocabulary the naturalistic child has a fairly distinctive and predictable pattern in giving definition to words. The naturalistic child thinks in a "holistic" and visual pattern. This means that if we ask a child such as this the definition of a word like "rake" that we will get a one word perceptual response such as leaves, move things, or pick up. He will be describing what he "sees" and this will often involve the behavior, the use, or the essential characteristics of the word meaning but little or none of the elaboration in a description. Further, the child will often stumble for words or simply say that he does not know. In this case if we press the child we can obtain a great deal of information including the fact that the child knows that the rake is a tool, an implement, or some other generalization, which yields a more complete answer. This often transfers to the classroom where the child has difficulty finding the words to express himself.

e. On the general information subtest these children often surprise us if not with complete descriptions at least with the amount of fragments of information they have about social values, about practical solutions, or common sense answers. General information requires such knowledge and the naturalistic child, with his keen awareness of nonverbal behavior and meaning, often is quite aware of why people do what they do, and possesses general common sense. Common sense implies an ability to see the basic reasons and purposes for things. The naturalistic child, with his high creative and insightful behavior, is quite aware, but he may have trouble expressing it.

f. When these children are asked to repeat a series of numbers they quite often do very poorly, because they drop the last numbers in the sequence, reverse the order of numbers, and generally have much difficulty. This is also seen in sequential classroom tasks like spelling, although these children, with visualization skills, can do well in spelling at least for the test. Their later recall, however, is quite poor. They will often stumble completely when writing a word in a sentence which the day before they seemed to know quite well for the test.

g. In tasks such as picture completion on the WISC-R, as in word attack skills and spelling, these children often attempt to view the entire or holistic aspects of the visual structure and miss specific details. With some urging they can see specifics, but often their general eye movements are designed to serve the gestalt hemisphere rather than the digital and sequential left-to-right needs of language structure. Forcing the child to use his finger to assist visual search often eliminates the tendency to scan and miss detail. In this way the specific analysis in visual tasks, though seemingly a spatial task, is often more influenced by verbal-sequential organization.

h. Picture arrangement on the WISC-R consists of a series of pictures that must be arranged in an appropriate order by the child. Many reading exercises in today's materials also utilize this sort of task. Because the task involves the use of left to right sequencing and order many researchers see this as a left hemispheric or digital task. Further, many researchers see the verbal directions as implying a great deal of left hemispheric input. This is all generally true but misses the actual function in right hemispheric organization, in which spatial tasks must be organized in a sequential and directional organization. To assume that because sequential organization is required left hemispheric input is involved is too simplistic. This is a partial interhemispheric task but can be a totally nonverbal one. Our own work with some 4,000 children indicates that high right hemispheric children often do exceptionally well on this task. Further, an excellent indicator of the directional errors of the spatial child is his tendency to make the correct sequence but in a right-to-left pattern. As he concentrates on the nature of the sequence he inadvertently returns to a right to left orientation of the spatial hemisphere and organizes the sequence in that manner.

i. Block design on the WISC-R includes, again for many researchers, a great deal of verbal input. Yet, it is with block design that some of the most significant spatial assets and liabilities of the child are recognized in the manner in which he approaches the task. Given with typical standardization many spatial children *score* poorly on this task, but this is because of directional difficulties and due to timing. But the manner in which the child approaches and solves the task, without time limits, gives us the most important indicators of this task. Manipulation of the designs in this task involves mental imagery production of a special sort. In creative thinking, for example, one of the skills involved is that of transformation. This is the ability to look at a special design or an object and manipulate it mentally into different perspectives and positions. This ability allows us to make changes and predict outcomes of changes without actually making the changes. This is a highly spatial and creative task, most often associated with right hemispheric function. The left hemisphere can visually recognize similarities in design, but the execution of changes in that design is best accomplished through right hemispheric function. The highly verbal child with average or below spatial abilities tends to attempt to solve the design task by systematically trying various combinations. The highly spatial child often manipulates the possibilities in internal imagery and then puts together the design without trial and error. But often the spatial child will have difficulty in the directional orientation of the construction of the model and have to reverse parts of the design after making it. Yet, the spatial child approaches the whole task from a predictive mode.

j. The object assembly or puzzle task on the WISC-R is often one that spatial children do well. They enjoy its challenge, and parents often report that spatial children enjoy puzzles of all sorts. Again, highly verbal children often attempt to place the pieces together in a trial and error approach, while the spatial child perceives the whole of the task and performs it without hesitation once a spatial concept is formed.

k. The digit symbol task involves speed and fine motor skills and most often the spatial child has difficulty with this task not so much because of inability to remember different number-symbol relationships, but because of difficulties in directional and fine motor skills along with the factor of speed.

These specific areas of interest on the WISC-R, while important in each case, are only valid in recognizing the high spatial child when several indicators are evident and when combined with other data already suggested. Other factors, within both diagnostic and educational situations, are also very important. A summary of educationally related factors will be presented shortly, but some additional comments need to be made about actual diagnostic situations.

The approach spatial children demonstrate to the WISC-R items is often an interesting one. They often show little interest if not outright disinterest in verbal items, but their attitude often changes when they take the spatial portion. That they enjoy these sorts of tasks shows there is often a very different orientation, and the children show outright pleasure during the spatial testing. They see the tasks as games and this difference in attitude between the two portions of the test is important to observe, for it also reinforces probable spatial competency.

The high spatial child often has difficulty, as was mentioned earlier, in directional orientation. At times they organize from left to right, but sometimes they switch to a right to left orientation. This is due to the uncertain dominance they exhibit between left and right sensory motor areas. Even though the child is right-handed, there is often an ipsilateral control of the hand giving him a tendency to work and organize from right to left. This competition between the two hemispheres may go one way or the other, and sometimes the child simply organizes vertically, as in drawing tasks, and avoids the whole issue. An essential characteristic and consequence of this spatial confusion is a tendency to orient in time from right to left also. The child may end up reading words backwards or thinking about the sequence of numbers or days from left to right or right to left, with the result being that the words before and after become very confusing. Like the left-handed child who also has this difficulty, this child can eventually sort it out with practice and repetition.

It is the lack of good directional spatial-motor dominance that often creates so much difficulty in organizing this child's world. The cerebral tendency of the high spatial child tends to create directional confusion regardless of whether he is right- or left-handed. It is this spatial-cognitive relationship to spatial motor function that often is missed by the diagnostician. It is difficult enough to be left-handed or right-handed and left tending motorically, but the problem is compounded if the cerebral style tends to be one of spatial-creative orientation in the right hemisphere in addition.

If the child is spatial-creative, then his approach to problems, to time, and academic work will tend to be freeflowing and non-directional. It will be difficult to remember a sequence of directions, letters, or days in approach to learning or behavioral tasks. The child's orientation is one of scattered perception in which a problem or situation may be approached in any number of ways, as is so often the case with the creative child. He does not see a situation from the logical viewpoint, and he is unhampered by convention and logic, due to the strong influence and efficiency of the spatial hemisphere.

This directional and flexible orientation tends to demand that such children attend to the structure of letters when writing rather than to the content of what they are writing. In our earlier work we labelled this as a lack of motoric "automation," that is, the development of consistent and automatic fine motor skills in producing letter structure. Because they are often apt to make letters from right to left as easily as from left to right, they must constantly monitor their fine motor movements to assure they are producing the correct responses. This means they cannot concentrate on the content of what they are writing and must switch back and forth between content and structure. This results in poor attention to what they are writing and the actual production of the letters. This can often be resolved through repetitive drill and practice in developing automatic responses in written skills. This is not, however, only a problem for naturalistic children, it is one that is common with most of our culture when schools do not spend enough time on writing drill.

Communication Skills

The highly naturalistic child often experiences difficulty in language and communication skills. First, with his high spatial and creative intelligence and lesser language skills, he has difficulty talking while thinking through his thoughts at the same time. This is similar to the problem he experiences in writing, except more complicated. After all, the speech mechanism is also a motoric function, and it is primarily controlled by the language hemisphere. Since the naturalistic child's orientation directionally can be left to right or right to left, he has trouble sequencing his thoughts, which more often come as holistic units and integrated insights. In order to explain or communicate these large "chunks" of imagery he has to back up and slowly relate in sequence the nature of his thoughts. More often than not it is simply easier not to talk about his thoughts at all. When asked to do so he will experience everything from general confusion to stammering.

The highly spatial or, as we call him, naturalistic child is excellent at reading nonverbal behavior, which is in the realm of the right hemisphere. Thus, this child will often watch what a person does as much as listen to what he says. When the teacher gives a series of directions the child may be attending to her behavior, what she is wearing, or something going on outside the classroom. Once the other children begin to work, the child tries to watch them to gain some idea of what the assignment might be.

The naturalistic child often has much more imagery and ideational content than he is able to express, and this is why he needs much assistance in learning to communiate his ideas.

General Personality Style and Interpersonal Modes

The naturalistic child demonstrates many troublesome difficulties in personality and social relationships. It can be predicted that, due to his highly creative cognitive style, he will often be preoccupied with his own thoughts, and he is often seen as an egocentric child who does not attend to the needs of others. He can learn to do this, but when one is creative much attention is given over to personal orientation. In play he will often want other children to play his game and engage in activities in which he is interested. He simply is not consciously concerned about approval but rather engaging in his creative activities. He likes to play with other children, for play is the basis for much of his world. Yet, if other children do not want to play, he often simply ignores them or attempts to dominate them.

The naturalistic child needs much assistance in learning to attend to the needs of others, in seeing the effects of his behavior on others, and learning to follow directions in play which involves cooperative behavior. The naturalistic child will tend to enjoy playing alone and has to be encouraged to join with other children.

General Motor Development and Value Orientation

As might be guessed the naturalistic child often has some difficulties in developing adequate moral and value orientation. He tends to be impulsive and center on his own ideas and desire to experience sensory stimulation. It is often less a case of what is the right thing to do than it is will it be fun or interesting. His reasoning concerning the right and wrong thing to do often involves what and how it makes him feel rather than if what he is told is the proper thing to do. It is not that he is amoral, but he simply does not attend to social values so much since social values are part of the language structure which for him is not well organized. He may do something in the classroom or on the playground which hurts or in some way displeases another child and which may go against "good" behavioral standards.

But the problem is mostly the child's orientation to spatial organization and not that he does not care about being "good." One mother related a story which illustrates the point very well. Her ten-year-old creative daughter did not clean up her room when asked to do so. The mother became very angry at her and threatened her. Later the mother went into her own bedroom and found that the daughter had changed the room a bit and placed a picture she had drawn on her pillow. It was obviously an attempt to please the mother and she had spent much time apparently making the picture and doing some rearranging of items on her mother's dresser and other parts of the room. The mother was pleased until she went to her daughter's room and found it had not been cleaned. These children want to be loved and in fact are often very affectionate children, because that is the way they communicate. But in this case the child still had not followed directions. These children need an extra dose of explanation and reinforcement in learning good social values. Their level of moral development too often fixates at the instrumental level where things are done because there are rewards or punishments and not because they eventually internalize the verbal concept of right and wrong.

Intra-family Role and Interaction

The naturalistic child in the family is often the "bimbo" who forgets, is clumsy, gets into trouble for his creativity, and is emotional and impulsive, all resulting in a slightly antagonistic role within the family. Yet, he may be admired for his art, his music or athletic abilities, and his humor or childlike qualities. The parents are often frustrated at his inability to organize and his emotional outbursts. This can create difficulties for the child's development of an adequate self-concept and role in the family. The family often begins to excuse his behavior with the typical response of, "Well, what can you expect?"

Educational Implications in Research on Hemisphericity

The research on hemisphericity, while fascinating and often controversial to psychologists and others, reveals some relatively new insights into instruction and curriculum organization for schools. If we can step beyond the glamour of looking at the right and left brain as such and investigate the importance of hemisphericity in relation to learning and behavior, we move from the current interest in education to fundamental differences in how we look at children and how they develop. Becoming a bit more realistic we, as educators, must again come to the realization that too often what seems to be a revolutionary new theory is little more than additional information in how children develop. It may be new to us but the brain has been operating on the same practicalities for a long time. It is not so much that we have discovered a new frontier as we have removed another of the mysteries of ourselves. But what does all of this hold for school personnel? A great deal as we shall suggest here and illustrate in the case studies. The following potential insights must be considered and incorporated into educational technology.

Learning and development proceed not only on the basis of instructional opportunity but upon the natural organization and integrities of the central nervous system.

We have always known and given a great deal of "lip service" to the concept that children learn best with the use of concrete learning experiences first and then more abstract learning. Children seem to learn best first through gross motor experiences and then move toward more refinement and specificity in cognitive abilities. Stated in terms of hemispheric development, the brain first processes sensory data through "hands on" involvement with information and then proceeds to abstraction of that information through language abilities. In this sense, at least for learning in kindergarten and early elementary school, the curriculum must involve much activity-centered instruction, which is follwed by more verbal application. Let us use reading as a primary example of how we "should teach" utilizing normal central nervous system development and then look at what we do in practice.

Children first learn experiences with perceptual learning. They feel, taste, note the color of things, their texture, their measurements, and behavior. Following observing things and repeatedly testing them to see if they continue to do what they first do, the rolling the ball game, children come to expect certain things of the world. When the expectations become routine the child is ready to abstract and file away the information. This is done through learning the "name" of the thing or behavior. Then, with some practice, Tommy not only knows what you mean when you say "go to bed" he can now respond with a "no." So perception becomes abstracted in memory and can then be pulled out again with words. Eventually Tommy learns to recognize the words in printed form, which is another abstraction, and he begins to read. When he recognizes the words then he learns to write them, and education continues.

In this example we see first high nonverbal or naturalized learning in concrete form which is eventually abstracted into language and then finally into printed letters, which can be reproduced by the child. All of this illustrates the way the left and right brain work together to learn even at later ages. We all tend to revert back to tasting and touching when we are unsure about what we are seeing. Our naturalized and sensory processes always take precedence when we are learning something new or checking something out "for sure." The same is true in learning more complex information. For example, this concept not only implies a sequence of natural to verbal but also gross to refinement. In learning something new it is easier to begin with an "overview" of what we are to learn and then look at the various parts of it to truly understand "its workings." Again, gaining a holistic concept of something is an easier way to understanding because our effort makes more sense when we perceive the overall goal. It is our naturalistic and right brain that is able to grasp the whole of things and then our language hemisphere begins the process of separating out the parts logically to see the true nature of the whole. Only in higher learning and philosophy do we become more and more abstract in a sort of integration of part-whole learning where it is difficult to fathom the sequence of whole to part or natural to verbal. This concept then, based on general hemispheric function, sequence, and integration gives a key to the most effective way to teach all children. It speaks much about the process of teaching reading.

In reading we often teach children through verbal information without the prerequisite of giving them experience in what the words mean. Children constantly search for the "idea," the goal, or the whole meaning of a thing and too often the words give none of these unless we prepare the child. Adults usually learn similarly. This is the purpose of the outline of a course, the introduction in a book, and the listening to a song before we attempt to sing it ourselves.

Too often, then, highly verbal children learn the parts and miss the inference or the feeling while naturalistic children get the feeling and general idea but miss the specifics which are often important. It makes sense then that early reading must be a combination of experience and language, not merely word attack skills. This is why totally phonetic approaches fail with the slow learner or the naturalistic child. Conversely, the highly verbal child, learning the logical code easily, eventually is unable to create his own thoughts because they are tied to formulas and concepts given to him when he lacked the actual internal understanding and sensory insight into the words. Highly naturalistic children will require a language-experience approach while highly verbal children will learn best through phonetics. The children in between can learn best through combination approaches.

Different hemispheric styles will require different modes of information processing.

Not only must different children be taught reading differently, but the entire style of presenting information will need to be altered. For example, the highly naturalistic child will look for the visual and sensory aspects of a language experience while the verbal child will look for the logical and systematically organized aspects of the experience. The naturalistic child, after taking a trip to a natural setting such as a park, will remember all sorts of information about how things smelled, felt, looked and acted, but he may not remember even the name of the park, let alone the many other words that he experienced. The logical child, with his verbal and systematic mind, will recall his experience in sequence and name all of the places he has been. But he will often miss the more naturalistic aspects of the experience. Further, he will often remember what people said and did, while the naturalistic child will miss the people altogether in his egocentric experience.

The principle applies in the classroom as well. The verbal child will be able to remember lectures and take notes while the naturalistic child will remember the films, what the teacher put on the board, and the general idea but have difficulty with understanding what is said and with taking notes. This means that instruction must be both visual and verbal if the students are all to learn.

Each of these cases, the example in reading or the example here, will put either the visual or verbal child at a disadvantage. The teacher's task is to figure out how to present and teach in such a way that adequate opportunity for children to learn is provided.

Varying hemispheric styles will produce differences in behavior and personality. The teacher or adult has to work toward reinforcing the skills of the nondominant or atypical behavioral style of the child.

The highly naturalistic child moves a lot. He tends to miss the feelings and needs of others. He tends to enjoy fantasy and imagination and often is triggered into a period of daydreaming by some incidental thing in the classroom or his work. He pays little attention to sequence and forgets directions easily. The verbal child tends to organize well, to work toward perceived goals, to attempt to please others and worry about their opinion of him, and attend to a task over a period of time. Each of these children can present problems for each other and the teacher. The naturalistic child is disruptive while the highly verbal child is overly goal- and value-oriented. One is overly flexible and the other too disciplined. Both need to move in the direction of the other in personality and behavior.

The teacher's task, rather than labelling one child as chaotic and hyperactive and the other as compulsive and rigid, is to provide experiences in which both children can learn to be more complete in their general behavioral response styles. All of the children in the middle do experience both, but the two extremes often have difficulties in general social and personality skills. This is an area in which we spent much time in our book on holistic health for children. Too often we label the extreme children as emotionally disturbed or learning disabled when in fact they present different hemispheric styles of response and need assistance and reinforcement in learning to behave differently. Most behavioral problems are difficulties in learning, not innate or emotional problems.

These three brief principles and examples illustrate the broad implications of the hemispheric theory. But the essential point is that the theory gives us another way to understand specific learning in developmental terms rather than always labelling a child or teaching in a specific way because it is traditional or seems logical to us. It is not so much that we are concerned with the theory itself as learning another aspect of normal child development and difference. We will refer to these and other concepts as we discuss the case studies.

Implications of the Theory and the Need for Further Research

The concepts surrounding hemisphericity are continuing to develop within psychoneurological research and, as has been in the past, that research will eventually become integrated into the educational and child development literature with resultant effects on notions about instruction. Already many of the earlier notions about the clear lateralization of functions into the two hemispheres and resultant effects on learning and development are being questioned by additional researchers who are looking more deeply into the general concept of brain lateralization and function. What is believed today in this area already shows signs of being disassembled by additional research and insights. This is the reason that we are somewhat discouraged by the more liberal and progressive interpretations of left-right brain theory. Yet our discouragement is not because some are using a theory which, at this point, is still not well developed. Certainly, much of what is currently believed, particularly in education and psychology, will eventually come to be seen as too simplistic relative to actual brain research in coming years. But, as we have stated again and again, it is not the actual accuracy of the concept that is the point in applied technologies with children. If the present state of knowledge helps educators to look more specifically at how children learn and develop, even though specifics of the theory are inaccurate, then the needs of children will be served. We have too long ignored neurological theories and research in the field of education and relied on general concepts of instruction rather than relating those concepts to the actual developmental process of learning. As we look in a holistic way at the theory and begin to move toward more specificity, then with additional research we can refine and alter our ever-deepening understanding of children.

Our greatest problem is to discourage the wholesale purchase of the theory as a new panacea and encourage educators to look at children, consider the theory, and walk cautiously forward waiting for more data. Our second problem is to encourage psychoneurologists to consider the more practical implications of their research and communicate that information to educators and psychologists who work with children. The distance between psychoneurological theory and the elementary classroom is so great that this may be difficult. It behooves educators and psychologists then to search out new information and work to apply that between fields. The psychoneurologist's task is formidable, but his is not the problem of applying information to the field of education. Rather, it is primarily the task of psychologists and educators to learn what they can and accept that theirs is the task of application.

We use the theory then as a general model, a practical way of looking at development and the system that supports it. We talk in terms of right and left hemispheres, and yet we know that in fact there is no such clear and definable process within the human brain. This is only a means of getting a hold of the theory in order to make it fit into our system of instruction, to reorder our priorities and approaches. The central nervous system capacity for change and flexibility is awesome, and there is so little understanding of its function that we are less than pioneers, we are blind people groping in a world in which we barely understand the essentials. We must maintain an open set of concepts, apply them as we can, and observe and evaluate the efficacy of the results.

Chapter 3
CASE STUDIES — GROUP A

IN the following discussions we want to explore the various aspects of the hemisphericity theory in relation to problems children exhibit in school and in personality. Before we can begin some general statements concerning various tests and procedures should be presented for those teachers who will be reviewing this material. Most of our discussions will involve the more practical aspects of the theory in relation to classroom learning difficulties. Psychologists who may also be reading the material may often wish for more clinical data. Unfortunately the purpose of our discussion is that of educational application, and an in-depth discussion of the more clinical factors is not appropriate. However, the psychologist should gain enough information to see implications for testing and some inferences can be made concerning clinical factors. It is important though that the concept of hemisphericity be given over to the practical aspects rather than the theoretical. The first case will be used as an overall example of how these children are evaluated along with some explanation of the tests used. Following the first case, less discussion will be provided concerning the actual tests used.

Case Study 1

Name: Sean
Age: 11-4, Fifth grade
School Setting: A small rural school with a traditional philosophy and a phonetically based reading program. There were thirty-one children in Sean's fifth grade class.

Home Setting: Both parents live in this middle income home with Sean and his seven-year-old sister.

Development: Sean walked at the usual age of about one year and developed language at the appropriate time. He has always displayed a high activity level, and during his sixth year it was discovered that he had an overactive thyroid for which medication was administered. Since this did not seem to help his hyperactivity, he was then given Cylert®, a similar stimulant to Ritalin®, which in turn did not seem to assist in reducing his overly active behavior pattern.

This case illustrates one of the common problems we see with many children; medical, psychological, and educational personnel often do not communicate well; critical information, along with many valuable insights into the child's needs, is never discovered, and sometimes treatment is administered needlessly. Yet, this is a continuing problem and one that is not likely to be resolved in the near future due to the difficulties in getting these professionals together with their many conflicting schedules and responsibilities. In this case we will see how important interdisciplinary communication can be.

Aside from Sean's hyperactive behavior he also has difficulty waking up in the morning, and he enjoys staying up late at night and working on the many projects that he builds in his room. He has purchased an old motorcycle and is rebuilding it in the garage. While he cannot bring the cycle parts into his room he brings many pieces into the house until his room is a collection of bits and pieces and nearly completed building projects. He never seems concerned about the mess and continues on despite his mother's protests. Sean has a good sense of humor which is also typical of children who have more efficient spatial organization than verbal.

In school, Sean has one of those teachers who has spent many years learning that children need discipline and responsibility. Sean is the bane of her existence, because he is constantly out of his seat and about the room. Even though she takes a rather punitive approach to him he seems not to mind and simply smiles and tells her how much he likes her. He often brings her small presents, most of which are not appreciated. She becomes so distressed at times that she sends Sean to the office. His cheery attitude toward others bewilders the teaching staff who, try as they might, cannot seem to get him to accept "responsibility." At one point the teacher isolated him in the room by placing sheets of cardboard around his desk. Much to her dismay he made a semi-truck design on the outside of the cardboard and soon had all of the other children playing in "his truck." The teacher scored 0 points while Sean scored 5!

Sean had much early confusion in determining left and right orientation. He continues to bat with the right hand and catch with the left hand, although he is predominantly left-handed. We often see this in children with cerebral dominance confusion. In that they have difficulty determining a dominant hand, they sometimes resolve this by using the left hand for some activities and the right hand for still different activities. Sometimes parents and teachers will see the child as ambidextrous when this is not actually the case. Few children, none that we have ever seen, are actually ambidextrous. The term implies equal abilities in both hands, which is neurologically improbable due to the fact that bilaterality enables us to divide the tasks cerebrally and designate one side or the other as the dominant side. The establishment of a dominant side provides one of the significant keys to our intelligence. We have first the division of labor, and secondly we have a definite reference point in space to determine left and right directional orientation. Without such a stable reference point we will be continually confused about which way is which. We must remember that the left-handed child uses a right-to-left orientation, while the right-handed child uses a left-to-right orientation. When a child does not establish a permanent dominant side he will often have difficulty remembering which way to orient. If the child is left handed, or right cerebrally dominant, while he will have a tendency to work right-to-left, the error remains internally constant and he can eventually learn to reverse the orientation. But children who do not establish such dominance are constantly in a state of confusion.

Sean is such a child, and while his parents and teachers merely see him as a child who is ambidextrous, in reality he is a child who has learning difficulties which eventually will result in a learning disability.

Sean's WISC–R scores are quite revealing, though not as dramatic as other children we will discuss. The following scores were achieved by Sean:

WISC–R:

Verbal:
Information – 8
Similarities – 8
Math – 9
Vocabulary – 9
Comprehension – 11

Nonverbal:
Picture Completion – 11
Picture Arrangement – 11
Block Design – 11
Object Assembly – 13
Coding – 8

Wide Range Achievement Test (WRAT):
Reading – 3.5
Spelling – 2.8
Math – 4.8

Peabody Individual Achievement Test (PIAT):
Reading – 4.2
Comprehension – 4.7

These scores are scaled scores and in the coming discussions the teacher should realize that scaled scores of 9 to 11 are considered in the average range, while scores of 7 and 8 indicate below average function and scores of 12 or more are in the bright range. The full range of scores goes from 0 to 20 with the retarded scoring below 6 and gifted usually scoring above 14 or 15. Again, for our discussion here we are not so concerned about the actual I.Q. score as we are the general concepts. In Sean's case an I.Q. score does not reveal much, for his verbal I.Q. is between 90 and a 100 or about 95. This places him in the low average range but not significantly. In spatial or nonverbal intelligence he has a score of 105 or in the 100–110 range. The average range is, of course, 90–110. Thus, in Sean's case, we see nothing unusual in his general intelligence scores. But when we look at specific subtest scores many things are revealed, particularly when we look at his behavior and work in school.

The first important factor to observe is that excluding Sean's above average or high average scaled score in comprehension, his information and similarities scores are very low. If all of his verbal abilities were this low he would be functioning in the slow learner range or below the average range of intelligence.

Information involves recall of specific information such as dates, names, or other practical and school-related data. Recalling specific information is often more difficult than recalling general information, for it involves a more finely tuned memory search. In our experience, auditory memory, specifically digit memory, is very dependent upon spatial organization. Much of our memory structure is spatially organized, that is, we tend to "look" for it, and there seems to be a visual-spatial relationship between one's specific auditory memory and one's spatial competencies.

Sean, as many children with directional and spatial difficulties, has trouble with specific recall. This takes us back to the developmental and organizing principle that naturalistic development precedes verbal development with verbal organization being somewhat dependent upon sensory and spatial experience.

We see many children like Sean who are assumed to have a language disability when in fact the problem lies more in poor spatial organization. Verbal information goes into the system but it is not organized and it is difficult for the child to "find" or retrieve it on command. In Sean's case giving him multiple choice questions following the standardized questions often revealed that he could "recognize" the right answer but could not retrieve it. There are children who are language deprived and who suffer a lack of learning and experience. Such children do not "know" the answer and therefore we are dealing with real language problems.

Sean was therefore having difficulty primarily in directional orientation due to poor cerebral dominance. This resulted in poor directionality, in a lack of dominant handedness, and in a tendency to orient sometimes to the right and sometimes to the left. He learned to use his right hand for some activities and his left for other activities. We have found that very bright children can sometimes achieve this because they have adequate conceptual ability to compensate for the directionality difficulty. But Sean does not have high language or performance abilities, and thus the directional problem interferes greatly with his overall learning efficiency.

Another factor in Sean's case is that he not only has slightly higher abilities in nonverbal areas, his general personality structure is centered around activity, or sensory information, for this is the easiest sort of information for him to use. The fact that he lives in the country and deals with mechanical things also tends to reinforce additional interest in nonverbal learning.

Sean's poor language skills, along with his nonverbal interests and experience, make it difficult for him to sequence time well, and often he does not pay attention to cause and effect. He focuses nonverbally on mechanical things and less on listening to directions or organizing his behavior into appropriate sequences. This adds to his overall distractability for verbally related items but does not affect nonverbal function. If something comes into his head, and it often does, he will set out to explore it, forgetting for the moment whatever task he is about. This happens continuously in the classroom as he is distracted by noises, colors, and even thoughts that happen to come into his mind. We usually hear those random thoughts called "day dreaming." Actually the day dreams of nonverbal children are much like the organized problem-solving mental activities of the verbal child. The nonverbal child simply "thinks" in visual images and constructs or plays out ideas in his head. It is not so much simply drifting about aimlessly in his head, which is often the nature of day dreaming, as it is creative thought. Sean tends to drift into creative thoughts easily and cannot stay on task.

In Sean's case then we have several important factors that need to be listed concerning his cognitive and personality style:

1. Though there is little difference between verbal and nonverbal intelligence, Sean's language is depressed adequately to provide enhanced experience for him in the nonverbal mode.
2. Sean's personality and experience tend to reinforce his nonverbal tendency.

3. Sean has difficulty with dominance and continues to have some confusion concerning left and right orientation.

4. Sean has poor language organization skills, particularly in specific recall, abstraction, and vocabulary. This results in difficulty organizing his attention to verbal tasks and difficulty retaining a conscious orientation to the follow-through of those tasks. Yet, his nonverbal abilities and his interest in spatial-motor tasks is high average to above average. He therefore can be expected to have difficulty in organizing verbal tasks and will tend to drift to imaginative or nonverbal mental activities.

5. Due to his directional difficulties and his poor language organization ability, Sean has poor fine motor skills. This complicates his problem, for even when he does pay attention, his writing is so poor that he becomes discouraged, which again causes him to avoid the task.

With these difficulties in mind we can proceed with an additional analysis of Sean's difficulties. In point number 5 above, a common problem is seen in children who have a cerebral difference with spatial abilities being higher. There exists a type of cerebral competition between the two hemispheres for control of the hand. Though Sean is left handed his dominance in motor function is not well established. Thus, both motor areas may have input to motor function and cause some competition in making fine motor decisions. A well-organized left-handed child can learn to reorganize his movements in the opposite direction relative to internal feelings. But if there is poor dominance then there are tendencies to work both directions causing great difficulty in fine motor function. The gross motor functions such as throwing, catching, batting, or activities of strength can be managed, while fine motor movements requiring high degrees of control and execution may be severely confusing. Such problems will create writing and spelling problems. Yet, the child may be able to draw adequately, for there is a great deal of difference between creative fine motor expression, which comes from "within," and recreating fine motor symbols that must be duplicated from external models such as letters. When working from within, such as drawing a picture, the child can begin at any point and go in any direction he chooses. But when making letters he has to make specific movements designed by someone else. In the second case the competition becomes apparent and the child has great difficulty. This is a significant problem for Sean.

The execution of fine motor skills according to external models, when there is poor dominance or competition, becomes a difficult problem for the child and can be resolved either through much practice in fine motor skills or through repetitive drill in letter structure. This can often be accomplished if such drill is introduced when the child is five or six years old. The fine motor skills are practiced to the point that they become automatic. This means that the child no longer has to monitor his movements and can concentrate on "what" he wants to write instead of "how" he is writing it. If the child does not develop automatic writing skills or, as we term it, "automation," then during writing activities he has to continuously "switch" his attention from what he is writing to how he is writing. During such switching processes he may forget part of what he is writing. This shows up particularly in spelling where the child drops letters, reverses the order, or inserts letters that are not in the word. Ask the child to spell the word verbally and he may have no difficulty. But during spelling tests he may misspell many words simply because he is not "aware" of the dropping of letters or the reversals. He "thought" of the correct spelling but inadvertently did not write all of the letters because he had to focus his attention on making each letter.

This is a common problem for many children when they are not given adequate instruction in writing and are not given time to truly develop an automatic skill. In cases like Sean's, or the child with high hemispheric function in spatial abilities, this is a very frequent problem. In most cases both normal children and special children can be spared the frustration if good teaching procedures are followed. Too often today, few schools really provide an adequate writing program in either manuscript or cursive writing.

Creating Dyslexia

Sean is a prime subject for producing dyslexia as a result of the misunderstanding of his developmental needs and a lack of appropriate instruction. In the authors' viewpoint the term dyslexia should only be used with children who have remarkable inability to associate visual symbols with sounds. This is a very rare disorder. In most school programs today children are given the label of "dyslexia" merely because they have severe reading difficulties. Often this label also carries the implication that the problem is constitutional and has nothing to do with instructional methods or classroom technology.

In the school's definition of dyslexia several characteristics are commonly observed to earn a child the label. The following list is typical, although certainly not inclusive, of all the characteristics invented by educators:

1. More than two years behind in reading achievement in relation to mental age.
2. Tendency to reverse letters and the sequential order of numbers or directions.
3. Poor fine motor skills.
4. Distractability.
5. High level of motor activity.
6. Difficulty learning phonetic sounds.
7. Poor short-term memory.
8. Impulsivity.
9. Emotionality.
10. Poor writing skills.

A quick glance at this list tells us one important thing, educators and many psychologists are confusing the medical classification with behavioral and learning traits of children. It is true that most dyslexic children will demonstrate some, if not all, of these characteristics. But it is also true that as many as 30 percent of *all* school-aged children will exhibit these same characteristics. Something is wrong, for the actual incidence of clinical dyslexia is probably less than 1 percent if that high. And in our last sentence we let the educational cat out of its proverbial bag. Clinical dyslexia is used by clinicians to make a differentiation between what is commonly referred to as dyslexia and the actual existence of neurologically defined dyslexia. In clinical dyslexia there are neurological indicators which point to a significant central nervous system impairment and prevent normal ability to associate visual symbols and sounds. Developmental dyslexia is also used to designate children who have severe problems in reading. But these problems which are caused by difficulties in specific developmental abilities, most often can be resolved or remediated through educational intervention. The list just given is typical of developmental dyslexia. We usually avoid the term altogether and simply say the child has developmental differences or difficulties which interfere with learning to read, unless the child has verification of significant neurological problems.

In clinical dyslexia, special education intervention is usually required and even then the success rate is very poor. Most often the child has to be taught by auditory methods with only minimal reading skills ever being achieved. In developmental dyslexia the story is much more interesting and applies to Sean.

Most of the developmental dyslexia cases we have seen are associated not only with a child's poor developmental abilities, but most significantly with the educator's lack of understanding of child development and subsequently attempting to teach a child through methods inappropriate to his needs. In this sense the teaching methodology is as much a part of the creation of the so-called dyslexia as is the child's unfortunate difficulties.

In Sean's case with the many difficulties he is experiencing "developmentally" the worst possible method of teaching reading is through a phonetic, part-to-whole, approach. This, of course, is the method being used. With Sean's difficulties in language, poor sequential abilities, directional confusion, high interest in spatial and structural information, and his lack of interest in specific verbal information, along with poor short-term memory for information, it should be obvious that phonetics would be difficult if not impossible. Are there adequate alternates?

The answer to the question is a definite yes. Before discussing what was done for Sean let's mention some of the additional tests that were given to Sean, which will be discussed at various points in coming discussions. We mentioned the WISC-R and additional comments will be made on that test. The new Kaufman test will be part of the same battery of tests as the WISC-R and must be used by a trained psychologist.

For drawing Sean was given the Berry Developmental Test of Visual Motor Integration. This test is a drawing test that includes many forms that the child has to copy. It gives a good indication of the child's overall fine motor skills and can be given by a classroom teacher, though most often the psychologist uses this test. A similar but more complex test is called the Bender Gestalt and it should, in most situations, be given only by the psychologist. The Wide Range Achievement Test is commonly used by psychologists to measure reading ability, but it can be used by the classroom teacher. The problem with this test is that it is only a recognition test and includes both spelling and computational math tests as well. It is a good screening device but does not tell much about actual reading skills. On the WRAT, as it is called, Sean achieved a reading grade equivalent of 3.5, spelling of 2.8, and math of 4.8. Poor as this achievement is for a fifth grade boy, it is higher than his actual in-school reading level. In the classroom Sean is reading little better than late second grade. For obvious reasons the recognition test on the WRAT does not tell us how well Sean can read by himself in the classroom, his endurance, comprehension, or his ability to get his work on paper. For these reasons the teacher and the psychologist must be careful about accepting test results unless the actual nature of the test used is understood. Another test, the Peabody Individual Achievement Test (PIAT), is also used by psychologists and can be used as well by the classroom teacher. It is primarily a recognition test and involves having the child look at pictures or words and point to the response asked for by the examiner. For example, in reading comprehension it gives the child a sentence which he must read and then he has to pick out a picture which displays the meaning of the sentence. This is a very good test but has the problem of eliminating the child's need to verbalize and synthesize the information. He only has to recognize the correct visual representation of the sentence content. Again, this is a good test and includes both reading recognition and comprehension along with other subtests, but it also tends to score the child's skills higher than they would be in the classroom. On the PIAT Sean scored 4.2 on recognition, and 4.7 on comprehension.

The question which arises here is why did Sean score so much higher on the second reading test than the first? To understand this we must look at how Sean attempts to read, regardless of how he is being taught. This will also illustrate why sometimes inappropriate instruction causes a dyslexic-like condition.

Sean, like high right hemispheric children, tends to utilize a high spatial mode of perception rather than a sequential and verbal mode. He attempts to look at words like pictures, at the whole configuration, and uses both the general configuration and such cues as salient characteristics (the two "t's" in little or the two "o's" in look), prefixes or suffixes, or other distinctions. In this sense he does not "see" the word but only specific characteristics. He most naturally utilizes an approach such as whole word or even more linguistic approaches rather than looking at the sequence of sounds and "logically" working it out. Thus when responding to the first test he has only the word to use but in the second test he is presented with visual pictures. By looking at the words or even part of the sentence he is able to figure out the correct response. He can use his high visual mode.

Sean should be taught through a whole word and a language experience approach, because this more nearly fits his cognitive-perceptual style of reading. Had the school understood this, and approached Sean in this way, he could have later learned phonetics once he had developed a sight vocabulary and basic reading skills.

For Sean school did get better. He was willing to work on cursive writing skills. The teacher worked harder at structuring his school experience and gave him more time on assignments. Where possible the teacher altered some of his work so that his assignments were shorter or he was able to verbally report his work. His reading program was changed to also include a more linguistic program using word families, similar word groupings, and many language experience stories to take advantage of his good imagination. From his own stories he developed more effective language skills and his syntax in expression improved.

Sean's parents were given special work for him to do at home to reinforce reading skills, and they spent much time having him read out loud to improve fluency and expression. Sean also had a tutor who worked with him in order to increase individualization.

Sean responded well to the increased attention and though he still becomes confused at times with directions and specific recall, this area improved greatly through learning study skills and better methods of preparing for tests. These children often have to be given much repetition and practice in studying for tests. They feel they know the material because they understand it when they hear it. They subsequently do not study and then do poorly on tests. They have to be given much attention and parents have to help them organize their work and repeatedly study a particular lesson. These children do not usually rebel when someone "helps" them. They do rebel when they are told to study without help, and they find the organization and memory tasks overwhelming.

In this first case we have a child who, though not displaying significant hemispheric difference, displays some of the typical problems of a right hemispheric child through a combination of minor hemispheric differences and personality characteristics. This case is less complicated than others but illustrates many of the general diagnostic and educational problems.

In coming case studies we will explore many facets of the hemispheric difference syndrome. It is a complicated problem and there are no specific guidelines that resolve all cases. It is rather a matter of utilizing general concepts and then being creative in the diagnostic and educational analysis of the child's needs. We have found that the majority of children labelled learning disabled are really children who demonstrate developmental differences that are neither recognized nor understood. The worst indictment is when the teacher, unable to obtain the needed achievement from the child, reacts in frustration, accusing the child of being "unresponsible" or worse, a child with a severe personality disorder. Labelling, of course, does little good and looking within the child denies our own responsibility as teachers to participate in the child's development. The number of children labelled carelessly or because school officials did not have the needed developmental understanding is so significant that a new understanding of children is desperately needed. In the coming cases we will explore the many ramifications of the cerebral dissonance syndrome, but our discussions will touch on many aspects of the educational process which should be changed for all children.

There are some additional tests which should be mentioned before we continue with the following case studies. One test which is commonly used by both psychologists and teachers is the Peabody Picture Vocabulary Test. This is a test which has been used for some years and gives a verbal I.Q. score. The test is very short and for general purposes correlates well with other measures of verbal intelligence such as the WISC-R. Clinically there would be some argument with that statement but in the classroom the PPVT does give a good general indication of verbal intelligence. The test is not without limitations though, and the teacher should understand these before we use data from the PPVT in our case studies. The PPVT, like the PIAT mentioned earlier, gives the child verbal input from the examiner and visual data to respond to. There are a series of pictures in the PPVT and for each vocabulary word asked of the child, he must respond by pointing or saying the number of the picture. In this way a child is supposed to demonstrate his intelligence, since he does not have to verbally formulate his answer but merely recognize the correct response. Thus, the PPVT tells us much about what the child recognizes but not what he is able to actually recall and organize into a verbal response. Thus, the verbal intelligence scores on the PPVT and those on the WISC-R, while both may be within the same general level, communicate very different aspects of so-called verbal intelligence. It is important for teachers to recognize this. For example, with the highly right hemispheric child there could well be a tendency for him to score much higher on the PPVT than on the vocabulary subtest of the WISC-R. On the WISC-R the child has to formulate and recall responses. This requires a more complex spatial-verbal interface neurologically, while the PPVT requires a more spatial orientation without the internal imagery structure required in the case of the WISC-R. Both sorts of information have utility and merely because they are different does not indicate that one is preferred over the other. It is important that both the psychologist and the teacher recognize the specific nature of the various tests and how they can be used to recognize different learning styles.

There are many sorts of reading tests and those such as the WRAT, mentioned earlier, and one called the Slosson, are merely word recognition tests. The Slosson is also a verbal intelligence test, like the PPVT, that can be used by teachers to obtain a general measure of verbal intelligence. The Slosson also includes a word recognition and visual motor test.

There are few actual tests of performance for writing, and psychologists do not normally attempt to measure a child's skills in this area. Writing tests are available, but usually the visual motor tests along with having the child copy a paragraph from a reading comprehension test provides a good example of the child's general writing skills. Writing skills should be tested both while the child is copying and as the child does creative writing. This often gives a good indication of hemispheric difficulty in that the naturalistic child may copy fairly well but be unable to write at all when he or she is making up his own story. In some cases he is able to write his own story and do well in both spelling and penmanship, but it may take the child so long to do his work that it is impossible to complete it at school.

The following case studies will utilize some of these tests; when a different test or approach is used, such as a personality test, then we will discuss it during the case study. These general tests are most frequently encountered and will give us some framework of test data. The number of tests and procedures are multiplying daily, and about the country there are various tests that are favorites within a particular region. The cases we selected are those that are most likely to contain tests that are common throughout the country. We in no way intend to infer that these are the best tests or that they are the preferred ones. It is, rather, that these tests and studies were selected so that the problem of explaining the tests would not get in the way of the main issue of understanding hemisphericity. Any number of similar tests could be used to get the same information. But it is the technique and the knowledge of the examiner or teacher that brings to the assessment the critical insights. Given time to watch children in the classroom, much of the same information could be found by observing the children. In many cases those observations would be more accurate and realistic than what we get on our tests. Yet, the tests and the evaluation provide a shortcut to getting information and observing behavior. It is then the professional's job, teacher and psychologist alike, to make sense of the data they obtain.

Case Study 2

Name: Bob
Age: 7-2
Present Date: 7/15/81
Home Setting: Bob is the oldest of three children and lives with his natural parents in a small midwest town. His parents are self-employed. Bob's younger siblings are a new baby sister and a sister nearly two years old. It is often important, in a case such as this, to note that the first child was more than five years old before the arrival of the second child. In many respects then Bob was an only child until he entered school, or until the age when most children move on into school and become more independent from the home.

Developmental history: Bob had no significant problems during early infancy. He walked early, at about eight to ten months, but general language development was delayed. He spoke his first words at around 15 months but did not develop phrases until well into his third year. Following late speech and language development he still did not talk much and needed articulation therapy between his fourth and sixth years. He was always a shy child, slight of build and small for his age which was observed during his evaluation. He was uncertain of himself in social settings during preschool and continues to be a child who has a limited number of friends.

Temperament and personality: Bob is described as having a good imagination, liking music, and animals, and is often drawing at home. He likes gymnastics and is pretty good in this area. He learned to ride a two-wheeled bicycle at the age of five years and is generally well coordinated. He likes sports and is learning to play most major sports at his current age. Bob tends to get angry easily and then gets over it just as easily. He seems to be forgetful at home and, according to the parents, is somewhat disorganized.

Problems precipitating the Referral: Bob has poor reading skills, difficulty in following directions in school, and is restless along with having poor fine motor skills. The teacher feels he is immature and should be retained in the first grade.

WISC–R scores:

Verbal:

   Information — 6

   Similarities — 5

   Math — 9

   Vocabulary — 11

   Comprehension — 8

   Digit Span — 8

Nonverbal:

   Picture Completion — 16

   Picture Arrangement — 13

   Block Design — 12

   Object Assembly — 16

   Coding — 8

Verbal I.Q. score: 86

Nonverbal I.Q. score: 121

PIAT:

   Reading recognition — 1.4

   Reading comprehension — 1.2

Berry Developmental Test: 6.8

Draw a person:

   Conceptually adequate, perceptually poor.

Writing skills:

   Writing poor and large as is typical with younger children.

The foregoing information is adequate to provide a general basis for reviewing Bob's needs and development. Bob represents a special sort of hemispheric and developmental problem. Not only is Bob well developed and competent in nonverbal functions, but he is somewhat significantly underdeveloped in language abilities. But as we will see this first impression is not an accurate picture of his needs. His is one of those cases though where it would seem that we have a highly naturalistic child with high right hemispheric function. The problems are more complicated than this but this is the sort of situation that often faces teachers or psychologists. With a high spatial child shouldn't we expect certain characteristics to be true? Perhaps they are true, but what does one do now? At this point many of the advocates of right-left brain function really have little to say because their interest in the theory is to encourage creative behavior. Unfortunately, here is a child who is creative. What do we do with him, simply label him learning disabled? Let's explore the factors in this case and see where we go. This is not an unusual sort of situation and yet we often find teachers having difficulty understanding how to help boys such as Bob.

Overview of problem: In Bob's case we first want to note the significant differences between verbal and performance (nonverbal) portions of the WISC-R. This gives us an overview of his general organization. Next we want to see if he is left-handed and find that he is right-handed. We have then a child who may exhibit, remember we said may, some directional confusion due to the high efficiency of the right hemisphere and the use of the right hand. This can be a consequence of such a motor-cerebral arrangement. In Bob's case this is the situation. He likes to draw, play sports, and perform gymnastics, which are all related to high right hemispheric function. This verifies that the high naturalistic orientation is acted out behaviorally and in personal interests and preferences. We also find that he tends to be emotional, gets angry easily and gets over it quickly, has difficulty with time and organization, and generally displays the naturalistic pattern.

In our overview of the situation then it would appear we are dealing with a highly experiential and spatial child. Secondly, are there indications that the naturalistic tendencies are interfering with learning in expected ways? This would include poor writing skills, lack of interest and difficulty with phonetics and sequential organization, and poor organization in the classroom. Again we see the expected behavioral pattern of the high naturalistic child.

In some cases visual and whole-word approaches in reading, increased practice in writing, and assistance in organization within a well-structured classroom would be part of the recommendation. But in Bob's case there is a critical area of concern which complicates the situation. Bob has poor language skills.

We must turn our attention then to that aspect of the case. He already has a highly naturalistic tendency, and without at least average verbal abilities, he will be like a sailboat without a rudder.

He will be unable to control his attention or to benefit simply from these recommendations.

Bob's language skills are not, within themselves, low, nor are the intrasubtest scores consistently low. This complicates the situation more. Bob had terrible difficulty with the information subtest, that is specific recall of information. In this area he is functioning well below average. Why is this? In all of his language functions he has difficulty. A case like this usually arises from several possible causes:

1. Cultural deprivation in which there has been poor language stimulation.
2. Specific neurological or developmental delays for either genetic or situational factors.
3. Severe personality or emotional factors.

In Bob's case there is early developmental evidence of a significant language delay but neurological damage or insult is not verified and, if it were, it would not assist us much in solving the problem. There may have been some genetic or early insult resulting in the language problem but in that this cannot be changed we are simply left with the fact that there was an early delay. Cultural deprivation in this case is not acceptable in that the parents did provide not only an adequate language environment, but they gave good stimulation, were alert to his poor language development, and sought assistance early. There is no evidence of a severe personality disorder. In this case then we are left with the probability that even though there may be some neurological factors operating in early development, the best assumption is he needs assistance in the language area and that it may simply be called a developmental delay as was the situation in Sean's case.

But Bob does have very poor recall as well as difficulty in seeing relationships abstractly, i.e. the low score on the similarities subtest. These two areas, taken by themselves, represent a severe language problem. If all of the language scores were this low Bob would be functioning within the mentally handicapped range. But math and vocabulary are within the average range. Comprehension is low but again, this is an area of recall and common sense application requiring verbal organization. Our first critical factor is the low recall and abstraction difficulty.

Recall involves specific memory, and if a child has spatial-directional difficulties, i.e. poor fine motor and sequential abilities, he often has difficulty in recalling specific information. This was the case with Bob implicating a poor spatial structure. This then is related to his naturalistic tendency and hopefully some assistance in organization and spatial development will aid in the language deficit.

During the testing it was found that Bob could recognize the concept of abstract relationships if he was given the sort of thought pattern he should utilize. When given examples and some additional time, he was able to make the abstractions. Again, here are poor language skills complicated by a naturalistic organization. Yet, with assistance it appears that he could make the abstractions. Now instruction and teacher awareness of a child's needs are implicated in his problem. He does have poor language structure but without understanding the overall organizational structure of the child we might have inferred many other possibilities about Bob. Instruction can probably assist Bob if we go about it correctly.

Bob is a very shy child. This has not assisted the teacher in recognizing his needs either. He is quiet enough that the teacher sees, along with his general lack of independence and assertiveness, a great many learning problems and therefore she is correct in assuming that perhaps it is simply immaturity. Yet, just to repeat first grade probably will not resolve Bob's difficulty. He needs stimulation and special attention.

With the language difficulties and the high naturalistic function, as has been mentioned, there will be difficulty in fine motor and spatial-directional organization. Some of the problems resulting from this have been noted, such as poor recall and abstraction. At a very practical level Bob will suffer from a lack of writing "automation." That means he will have to attend to making letters due to his tendency to work in the wrong direction, and in order to make the letters there may be many structural errors. If we look at Figure 3 we see some of Bob's work on the

Berry Developmental Test. While normally done within specific blocks on a prepared form, we usually have the children simply copy the forms on a blank sheet of paper. The structured forms do not give us a chance to see how the child deals with organization and space in working with fine motor skills.

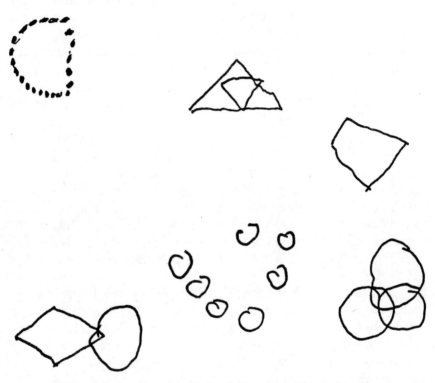

Figure 3. Portion of Bob's Berry drawings. (Size reduced.)

In Figure 3 several important factors can be seen that are typical of children with poor spatial-directional organization and automation difficulties. The forms are not placed in an adequate left-to-right fashion and are poorly formed. The typical child would place the forms left-to-right across the page. Bob, due to his difficulty in spatial motor function has to concentrate on the actual structure and is not able to consider the left-to-right orientation. In that he has to concentrate on structure, and it can be seen that his attempt is done very poorly, he produces inadequate reproductions, which are poorly organized on the paper.

This problem will be evident in writing and spelling activities. In writing (see Figure 4), though he is more than seven years old, there is much difficulty in reproducing the letters just as in reproducing the forms. The letters are large, indicating a lack of good fine motor control, spacing is poor, and the general organization is also inadequate. We can predict then that when Bob attempts to write while copying he will have poor understanding or comprehension of what he is writing, because he has to concentrate totally on the structure of the letters. Further, while copying is difficult, if he tries to write his thoughts on paper the difficulties will be more pronounced. Here he had difficulty reproducing the model, but when he also had to think of what to write he was not able to concentrate on both the content and the structure. The result is adequate thoughts with terrible structure and spatial arrangement, or, poor concepts and more adequate structure. Either way he will not be able to successfully work on any activity that requires written work. Further, he will be discouraged and this will contribute to day dreaming and an inability to complete independent assignments. This is the case and another reason that

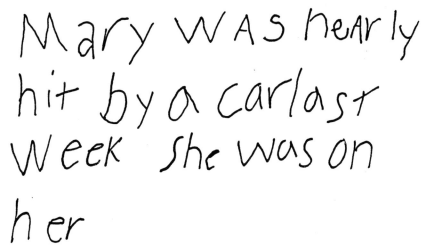

Figure 4. Example of Bob's writing. (Size reduced.)

the teacher sees Bob as immature. Actually he has developmental difficulties which will require specific assistance. Repeating a grade will not be enough in that it is not merely a case of immaturity.

With all of these factors in mind we can then formulate a general curriculum approach for Bob. Since Bob is shy and slight of build, along with his many difficulties, it may be appropriate to allow him to repeat first grade but with the following recommendations for the teacher:

1. Bob needs to be in a highly structured classroom where the teacher is sensitive to his emotionality, his need for support, and his tendency to become discouraged. Much emotional support will have to accompany the structure. Directions will have to be repeated, the teacher will repeatedly have to return to him during class to reorganize his efforts, and he will need to be given some additional time on written work.

2. Bob will need a program of writing development in which he practices individual letters on a blackboard with lots of space. He needs to spend much time making large movements and also the repetitive work of such writing programs as the "Palmer Method" or other such structured practice programs. Such work needs to be practiced until writing skills are automatic or can be performed without conscious attention to structure.

3. Language stimulation will be required in verbal expression, in syntax, sentence structure, and organizing thoughts. This can be combined with the following activity.

4. Reading skills need to be developed with as little phonetics and sequential structure as possible until his skills are better. This can be accomplished through a more visual approach in reading for the year. The whole-word or language experience approach would be most appropriate not only toward assisting him in reading but also in language development. Here we would ask him to make up short stories that would be committed to paper in typing or placed on the blackboard. He would read the words of his story, learn to recognize them through visual repetition, and through individual word analysis. We would teach him to look at structure and configuration, and look for prefixes and suffixes that occur

frequently. A linguistic approach utilizing word families, syllables, beginnings and endings of words, root words, and other such general principles would be introduced. This whole-to-part approach would be much easier for Bob to assimilate and at the same time assist in the development of expressive language. The parents should read to him at home and encourage him to reread stories with them without using phonetics but also using a whole-word approach.

In class Bob might still be enrolled and working to some degree with the regular reading skills such as phonetics. But this would not be given great emphasis until he developed more general whole-word attack skills. As Bob's general skills improve along with general organization, then phonetics should be reintroduced.

This brief overview of recommendations, according to our work, is usually very successful. It all demonstrates that understanding a child's development leads us to the sort of curriculum style and approach needed. Bob did respond well to the program. The next case to be presented displays a general profile similar to Bob's; poor language with higher spatial skills, poor fine motor skills, but the added feature of emotional difficulties and the trauma of losing a mother and gaining a step mother along with two step siblings. This next case illustrates how difficult it is to simply use the spatial or naturalistic syndrome to make an assessment of the child's needs. As we have mentioned, analysis requires a holistic viewpoint of each child looking for those important variables that will make that child's particular problems unique to only him, even though he may in many ways "fit" into a general behavioral learning pattern.

Case Study 3

Name: Eddie
Age: 7-7, Grade 2
Present Date: 1/19/81
Home History: Eddie is a boy who has suffered a most significant childhood trauma; his mother died when he was five years old. The father has since remarried and the new mother brought with her two children of her own, ages four and five years. Generally

Eddie would appear to have adjusted well, but there is evidence that things have not gone so well. One of the questions the parents sought in the evaluation was how to effectively "discipline" Eddie at home. The mother is also upset because Eddie does not adequately "clean" himself after going to the bathroom. Eddie tends to dominate friends and attempts to force them to play the games he wants to play. The parents also want to know why he tends to do things that they dislike. School achievement is not a significant problem, but he is not doing as well as the parents feel he should. The father is self-employed and the mother does not work.

Developmental History: Eddie walked late, taking his first steps at about 14 months, walking adequately by 18 months. He talked early, prior to the end of the first year, but his overall language development was not unusual in most respects. There were no unusual features about his development except for his tendency to dominate other children.

Temperament and Personality: Eddie is an assertive child who has had difficulty getting along with other children since preschool. He is an active boy and is always on the move. He tends to resist limits on his behavior and seems to have trouble learning from experience to correct his behavior.

While Eddie gives the impression of a fairly independent and assertive boy there is some evidence of personal uncertainty along with defensive behaviors to "hide" feelings of anxiety about failure and/or rejection from adults. There is evidence of anger toward adults, and it is postulated that he resents the new mother and particularly her two children. This is, for any child, a difficult adjustment, for it is hard for the step mother to prove her acceptance of the nonpaternal child as equally as her own children. Parents often need assistance in learning to recognize their own behaviors of rejection or acceptance of children in the blended family. It is felt in this situation that the mother was having trouble dealing with Eddie's behavior partly because of her poor understanding of his feelings and, her own inability to effectively show love and support. She too, had many feelings of rejection from Eddie and this contributed to the problem.

Problems Precipitating Referral: Eddie's difficulty at home was the primary problem for the parents, though his lack of good school achievement instigated their seeking assistance. Eddie did not get his work done at school. The parents were unable to assist him and many conflicts developed around school work. The mother was from a family of six children and the father was an only child. The father tended to take a lax management approach and was less concerned about Eddie's schoolwork than the mother. Further, the mother tended to be a disciplinarian while the father tended to give less importance to Eddie's behavior. This resulted in parental disagreements about management and tended to increase the resentment between the mother and Eddie.

WISC–R results:

Verbal:
  Information – 9
  Similarities – 6
  Math – 12
  Vocabulary – 9
  Comprehension – 10
  Digit Span – 7
Nonverbal:
  Picture Completion – 12
  Picture Arrangement – 13
  Block Design – 9
  Object Assembly – 14
  Coding – 11
Verbal I.Q. score: 95
Performance I.Q. score: 113
PIAT:
  Recognition – 2.3
  Comprehension – 3.1
WRAT: 2.1
DAP: Excellent
Berry: 6.8

The testing here would indicate several interesting factors in Eddie's general achievement and developmental abilities. We see an overall picture of a boy with generally capable naturalistic function and several difficulties in language function. Is his naturalistic competency so high that it is interfering with learning?

There is an eighteen-point difference between language and performance. That is fairly large and could be implicated in his overall functioning. But in this case there are obviously emotional factors, intrafamily difficulties, management problems, and learning difficulties. We would not lay all of this on the eighteen-point difference between verbal and performance, or naturalistic and socialized function. Yet, it probably plays a role. The concepts of hemisphericity do not give us a causal basis for many difficulties (though in some cases this may be true), but rather they are an important aspect for our understanding of a more complete picture. That is what this case has to demonstrate to us.

First then we look at overall organization and competency, language and spatial-creative function, and find that there is an interesting and perhaps important difference in these two areas in favor of nonverbal cognition. Let's look at each area briefly.

Eddie had difficulty recalling information facts but was not significantly poor. His math computational skills, though somewhat verbal in nature on the WISC-R, were above average. We will point out in many of the cases, though not always, that children with above average spatial ability conceptually often do well in math computation. Early math is a spatially oriented operation while higher math is more verbal. And here we have a boy who does have above average spatial ability. It makes "sense." He does well on simple computation problems but later on he may have trouble when math becomes more verbal, unless he becomes more linguistically organized.

Vocabulary was also slightly low but not significantly, and general comprehension was average. But abstraction was significantly low. Eddie is having trouble with abstract language relationships and generalizations. This is important for Eddie because he also has difficulty organizing his behavior and recognizing his responsibility at home and school. That fits with the difficulty in seeing relationships.

Let's explore this important area for a moment. Why would a child who had good early language and generally average language skills have such poor abstraction ability? Is he brain injured? Is it merely because he has such high spatial-creative organization? There is little general evidence of any specific neurological problem and we should be cautious with such a small difference in language-spatial abilities, to suggest the hemispheric function as a basis for poor language. He is not so creative that he ignores language function. It is specifically within seeing verbal relationships. How did he perform during the questions concerning language relationships? Here we find that he was able to recognize the relationships once examples were given. This means that the capability is there but he is having difficulty using it. Why?

If we look at the emotional environment *and* the difference in hemispheric patterns, then it may be that there is a tendency to avoid specific organization hemispherically and with some emotionality the problem is intensified. This seems to make more sense. If this is true then we have an important cluster of functions upon which to base remediation and assistance. He will need good organization from adults, lots of support, and consistency in behavioral management. This should help him *learn* to organize and see relationships using the capabilities he does have. Simply working on abstraction will not solve the problem. Eddie is very emotional, uncertain of himself, and continues to be hurt from the loss of his mother. It will take time to heal that and he must be given much praise and success both at home and school to assure that he slowly learns that he is O.K. and that he is able to perform and gain acceptance. The problem often involves the fact that he needs more than one school year to do this and even if he has a sympathetic teacher now any progress may be lost if next year's teacher does not follow up. Too often she does not because teachers do not communicate between grades very well. Further, the parents will need consistent and ongoing counseling to assure continued consistency in behavioral management at home over more than a year.

Eddie tended to be a very aggressive boy in early childhood and it is likely that this was reinforced by his father and natural mother. Now his step mother is a disciplinarian and is requiring that he accept responsibility and organize himself. That in itself, the change from a somewhat permissive environment for the first few years, to a highly organized environment, will take some time, for Eddie has to acquire new behaviors. And with the father and mother disagreeing it will be difficult for Eddie to accept new behaviors. Further, he is a sensitive and intuitive boy (due to his higher creative abilities), and he will probably be somewhat manipulative, often getting one parent to side with him, usually his father.

In spatial skills there is one area in which Eddie does not do well. He had a lower than average score in block design, which was much lower than his other spatial items. Why? The answer would be lost unless the examiner gave his test behavior on that item. He became frustrated with the designs and literally gave up. He was uncertain about how to do them and with some effort realized they were difficult and so he gave up. This failed him in this test, but it also avoided further evidence of failure for him. If he wanted he could rationalize that the test was too hard. It was not that he could not do it, it was just a "bad" test. Many children do this. We call it planned failure. It has the advantage of always putting off the final truth. Could he have done it if he tried? Sometimes it is better to purposefully fail than to risk trying and really failing. In Eddie's case, with his underlying uncertainty, this was a real possibility. His nonverbal intelligence would have made it possible for him to perceive this ploy even though he might not have thought it through. He has probably developed several "defense" mechanisms of this sort.

Let's look for a moment at Eddie's academic skills. There seems to be some inconsistency in his reading achievement. On the PIAT Eddie scored a 2.3 in recognition and a 3.1 in comprehension. It is unusual when a child scores higher on comprehension than on recognition. Why? In this case two factors are important. First, Eddie is a highly spatial child. Remember that these children can often recognize information though they can't remember it. On the PIAT Eddie did not have to read and remember verbal information. He read and then picked from VISUAL information the correct responses. Thus, he is able to recognize information visually better than he can actually read the words. Thus, on the PIAT he was able to get enough of the words to pick out the correct picture. In the classroom, as might be guessed, his reading comprehension is not as high as on this test. In the classroom he has to read and use verbal information and organization to select the correct response. His difficulties would be compounded by poor attention and general behavioral problems. In the classroom the teacher sees him as reading only in early second grade at best with significant problems in word attack skills.

Eddie has been the victim of another problem in education. When he began first grade he was exposed to Unifon following a kindergarten experience with early phonetics. He had enough difficulty with symbols and language but the two different approaches had left him more confused than organized and his word attack skills remained confused. In defense, and based on his natural tendency toward visual information, he attempted to read the whole word resulting in many whole word substitutions such as "felt" for "left" and "black" for "block." In that he was in a phonetic program in second grade, the school having dropped the Unifon program, he was having significant problems. Here we have a boy who should have had a language experience and whole word approach, struggling with two different systems of teaching reading, neither of which was the approach by which he could learn.

Eddie should be started on a language experience approach in order to stimulate the use of his imaginative abilities and to foster organizing his thoughts into concrete word structures. He could then learn to read his own stories after they are typed. Along with learning the whole word, prefixes and suffixes, looking at configuration, and practicing rewriting his story, the words could be used for spelling. Along with such an approach we would add basic linguistic skills including word families, similar sounding and appearing words, and other structural analysis. Syntax and general organization of sentences including some basic grammatical structure could be taught. He could also produce pictures to add to his story.

In Figure 5 we see a portion of Eddie's Berry Test illustrating some of his basic fine motor organizational problems. This particular part of the Berry illustrates poor overall mental organization resulting from high concentration on structure. Even though he concentrated on the structure the diamond is poorly formed as is the triangle. The triple crossed lines show a particular problem in production. Here he had difficulty in producing the diagonal lines which is common with children who have directional problems. As might be expected he has great difficulty with writing. In class then, Eddie is not able to produce his written work well and often is slow or unable to get his work done. This is more than a matter of immaturity, it illustrates a common problem in children with hemispheric differences like Eddie's. He will need much assistance in writing. He should practice some each day on basic strokes and care should be taken to assure that the needed organization and skill does develop. If this skill is not developed he will have continued difficulties, and later he will become more resistive to working on any written assignments.

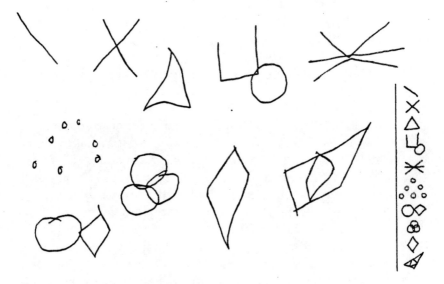

Figure 5. Example of Eddie's Berry. (Models shown at right.)

In Eddie's case then we have a number of problems including those listed here:

1. Emotional anger and stress as a consequence of losing his mother.
2. Difficulty adjusting to a new step mother and her more strict style of management.
3. Difficulty with management between parents who often fall into his manipulation of their behavior.

4. A tendency to dominate other children and difficulty seeing his own responsibility in behavioral situations.
5. Difficulty in language abstraction resulting in an inability to deal with his own behavioral organization.
6. Higher creative or spatial ability resulting in further avoidance of language and structure.
7. A lack of underlying self-confidence and an inability to recognize his ability to alter his own situation, to succeed in school and at home.
8. Confusion in basic word attack skills as a result of an inconsistent method of teaching reading.
9. A tendency to guess and use only whole word approaches.
10. Poor fine motor skills, although he has good artistic ability and skills.

These difficulties, as have been discussed, are all interrelated and must be seen as a whole in order to assist Eddie in resolution of the problems.

This case illustrates the problem of using hemisphericity as a single factor in a learning or behavioral problem. Approaches to the solution will require counseling the parents, stimulation in creative abilities, behavioral modification and management at home and school, reading assistance, assistance in organizing self-perception and social perception, and writing skills development.

In the following cases more extreme examples of children with hemispheric differences will be presented. These first three cases provide an overview of some of the problems in evaluating and using the hemispheric model. These cautions should be kept in mind as the following cases are presented.

Chapter 4
CASE STUDIES — GROUP B

IN the last chapter we discussed three cases that gave many of the basics for applying the theory of hemisphericity within an analysis of the problems children have in learning and development. In this chapter we want to explore other dimensions of hemisphericity, including both the blessings and problems of possessing high spatial abilities. In the final chapter we want to follow two cases over a period of time to see if specific intervention strategies work and how the differences in cerebral function affect them in the long run.

Case Study 4

Name: Tom
Age: 9-11
Present Date: 12/10/81
Home and School Setting: Tom is an only child living with his natural parents. He attends an open school where each student's program is individualized. The school is a small suburban school. Tom lives in a somewhat typical middle class housing development. The parents both work as bakers in a large commercial operation that has provided stable employment and allowed them to live somewhat comfortably. Tom is a "latchkey" child, arriving home from school about an hour before his parents arrive home from work. He lets himself into the house and there is a close neighbor whom he can go to if necessary.
Developmental history: Tom has had an unremarkable developmental history. He has always been a very loving child and the parents spend a lot of time with him. Some relatives feel Tom is

overindulged by the parents. He attended preschool and kindergarten and displayed no significant difficulties in either except that he appeared to need a lot of adult approval and attention. Teachers have described him as a quiet boy who seems too dependent and is not assertive enough.

Problems Precipitating the Referral: Tom is currently in the fourth grade and is experiencing some difficulty getting his work done. The teacher is a somewhat highly structured individual and even though the program is individualized, she expects each child to accept responsibility for his own work. Tom has found it difficult to work with so little attention from the teacher. The parents have been told by the teacher that Tom needs to be more assertive. The parents feel the teacher is not very supportive or sympathetic toward Tom, and they wish she would give him more attention.

In early October Tom began to complain of stomachaches and wanted to stay home from school on several occasions. Recently Tom had a complete physical examination, including a G.I. series, and no specific difficulties were found. The physician referred Tom for a developmental and psychological assessment.

WISC–R Scores:

Verbal:
    Information – 13
    Similarities – 11
    Math – 11
    Vocabulary – 12
    Comprehension – 12
    Digit span – 11
Nonverbal:
    Picture Completion – 15
    Picture Arrangement – 14
    Block Design – 15
    Object Assembly – 15
    Coding – 12
Verbal I.Q. score: 111
Nonverbal I.Q. score: 130

PIAT:
   Recognition – 3.2
   Comprehension – 3.6
WRAT: 3.0
Berry Developmental: 9-5
DAP: Simplistic but adequate.

    We should remind the reader that while in many cases other diagnostic data are available on each child only that information which is significant is included. In some of the future cases other sorts of information will be included. Our intent is not to present a complete diagnostic picture but to provide an overview of major diagnostic processes.

    Tom is demonstrating several factors that should be obvious to most people who work with children. Many of the characteristics here are "red flags" to a clinical psychologist. Tom is an only child, exhibited early dependency and a lack of assertiveness, has difficulty with school work, is a latchkey child, and has a strict teacher. It would seem obvious that here is a child who is reacting to demands that are too high along with an inability to meet the expectations without adequate support and love. The result, in classical psychological terms, is stress and anxiety expressed through physiological problems and complaints. In such a case it is not uncommon to tell the teacher she should be more supportive and the parents that they should receive family counseling. If this is done it should produce the needed support and understanding in addition to improvement in Tom's school work. That should end the drama.

    Unfortunately, most cases do not work out this simply and neither did this one. We could have found enough of family and child problems in this case to make for a long-term counseling case and it would have been beneficial to the parents. It would have also been time consuming and costly. In recent years, with the increase of knowledge about child development, we have found that there is little need for counseling on an ongoing basis with many children and families. One of the reasons is illustrated in this case. Most people, parents and teachers, can respond effectively in a short period of time to a child's needs if they are given concrete information that makes sense to them without instilling heaps of guilt. Sometimes the treatment creates as much stress and anxiety as the original problem and much of the time is spent "healing the guilt" of discovering one's mistakes. In this case for example, the parents could have been given a good dose of guilt over not being home to meet Tom which, according to general psychological theory, probably was creating much stress for Tom along with his other difficulties.

But, as will be seen, Tom's coming home to an empty house was not a critical part of his difficulty, and if anything, may have been an important responsibility for him. Let's delve into this case and see what holistic perceptions we can gain from the whole of the situation rather than from the traditionally obvious factors.

A little boy can be loving and need adult support. He can be nonaggressive and creative and not enjoy abrasive or competitive activities and be perfectly normal. Place such a child in the competitive world of nine to ten year olds, give him a teacher who expects little boys to be tough, and then instill him with a little difficulty in learning and we can "create" a neurotic child. At the outset of Tom's case we had to establish whether he was truly overdependent or if he was a more creative and sensitive boy who did not play the expected "male" child role.

At home the parents are fairly quiet people who enjoy classical music, who both paint, and who tend to be very demonstrative and loving parents. Whether it was genetics, environment, or both, they had created a little boy not unlike themselves. And it had all worked pretty well for them until Tom ran into Mrs. Jamison, the fourth grade teacher. But Mrs. Jamison was not a poor teacher, nor was she insensitive to children. It was a combination of factors that really did Tom in.

First, Tom is a boy who enjoys playing alone. He likes other children but is not assertive and does not enjoy the typical nine- to ten-year-old interests of most boys. He builds rather elaborate structures from wood and scraps and has a rich fantasy world. He has a Great Dane who has been his constant companion for many years and they are inseparable. He comes home to "Josh" and they often play while Tom is waiting for his parents. Tom is smaller than other children and is not very athletic. But he likes to play the piano and one day each week the teacher comes to the house when he gets home from school and gives him lessons. Another day after school one of his neighborhood friends joins him in a gymnastics class. The mother of his friend takes them and brings them home. While Tom does not like sports he does enjoy gymnastics.

Tom has always been a creative child and loves to listen to stories read by his parents from a "classics" series they bought for him last year. Someday he says he would like to write books.

If we look at Tom's WISC-R scores we see one of those typical "alpha" child profiles. He has a 130 nonverbal I.Q. with verbal abilities falling only in the upper average range. Tom tends to be somewhat impulsive and emotional. He is an expert with the Rubics Cube® and recently has become interested in computers. His parents bought him a small inexpensive computer, and he has mastered it and wants a bigger one.

Tom is right-handed but has always had difficulty with reversals and writing. His writing is not poor, but he has to work very slowly and this often prevents him from getting his work done on time. He is poorly organized in his work but is able to organize motoric activities, such as drawing and building, quite well.

When Tom's achievement scores are compared to his overall development, it is found that he is well over a year and a half behind chronological expectations and more than two years behind expectations for his mental age. In most schools today, Tom would be considered gifted in creative functions but only average in verbal abilities. He would not be selected for special gifted programs. In fact, his school has a program for gifted children. Sadly, it is for children who are doing well academically in school, and its goal is the development of creative abilities in bright children. Tom would love the program but he does not qualify.

Tom does quite well on the spelling tests at school, but when he writes creatively, spelling is not one of his priorities.

As we move along in our exploration of Tom his needs become more and more obvious when viewed from a holistic viewpoint. But there is more. Tom has severe allergies to food colorings and other substances which result in poor attention and irritable behavior. The allergies are under control through diet and medication. The teacher has often reported to the parents that he has somewhat severe changes in his behavior if he does not have his medication or, if the school lunch program includes something toxic to him. This, obviously, only complicates the problem.

When all of this information was reviewed by the teacher and the parents no one needed to feel guilty. Intervention was rather straightforward, and we might add, very effective. Following Christmas vacation there was a marked change in Tom's behavior and he no longer had the stomachaches or physical complaints. We apologized to the mental health and social workers who would have liked to make a neglect and dependent syndrome child of Tom. Again, analysis of behavior from a strictly mental health viewpoint must not continue as we discussed extensively in our book, *Holistic Mental Health for Tomorrow's Children.*

The intervention strategies taken in Tom's case include some very unclinical approaches, and even though he would have qualified for learning disabilities, he was never referred. This is typical of many cases we see where the data may indicate a significant difference between learning and developmental expectations and therefore rate the diagnosis of a learning disability.

One of the critical factors in Tom's case, even though the team had identified the major problems, was that of sequence and priorities. First let us list the major difficulties Tom was having.

1. The basic cause for referral included symptoms of stress, stomachaches, and Tom's unwillingness to go to school.
2. The stress was being caused by self-awareness of teacher expectations, by Tom himself, due to his high competency in spatial areas, and his sensitivity with lower verbal production ability. Tom wanted to do better and the teacher's expectations intensified this concern for him.
3. Underlying these emotional and social concerns were Tom's lack of fine motor skills related to writing and his difficulties in reading.
4. Underlying the lack of skills in writing and reading were difficulties resulting from hemispheric differences. The high spatial and average verbal abilities produced difficulties in the following ways:
   a. Directional uncertainty.

    b. Difficulty in using language skills such as sequencing, auditory memory, and recall of specific information.

    c. Tendency to look for whole-word structure rather than phonetic sequence.

The difficulties have to be approached from several points rather than attempting to resolve the underlying causes and working forward. Tom's stress had to be a focus of attention while at the same time making it possible to develop the needed skills which were primary in causing the stress. The following approaches were taken.

1. The teacher was advised that Tom would need much support in the classroom and that this could be accomplished in the following ways.

    a. The teacher would need to give Tom encouragement and let him know that she understood that he was frustrated.

    b. She would point out to him that she would assist him and that he would be able to improve some of his basic skills.

    c. The teacher would let him attempt seatwork in school, and leftover work could be taken home where his parents would help him finish.

    d. She would tell him that for a period of time some of his assignments would be shortened.

2. Tom was assigned to a volunteer teacher's aide three days each week where he was given blackboard practice for improvement of writing skills. One day each week he received typing instruction which would assist him in becoming more organized in his thoughts and help him to begin developing an alternate skill for expressing his ideas.

3. Tom was enrolled in a remedial reading class. In this class he was given assistance in whole-word analysis and linguistic approaches. He was also given language experience activities including his writing of stories with concern for sentence structure, syntax, progression of ideas, and basic grammatical skills.

4. The classroom teacher began to give Tom assistance in learning study skills involving scanning, outlining, and methods of studying for tests.

5. Tom was assigned to a school counselor who helped him set goals for himself each week. They wrote contracts together and this assisted Tom in seeing his own progress. This tended to make areas of difficulty less damaging in that he was able to begin to look realistically at both his successes and failures in a more balanced manner rather than overreacting to his failures.

The important point in this case is that too often many children experience difficulties that could be prevented if the teacher and parents understood the child's general personality and developmental make-up. What happened to Tom might not happen to another child who was less sensitive. The problems could have been predicted if there had been any reason for the teacher to make an in-depth analysis of Tom's school progress and his needs early in the school year. The problems could have been prevented if there had been some sort of realistic school developmental progress program for each child.

This case illustrates that a child with cerebral dissonance, though this creates a different emotional and intellectual style, need not become a problem for the child. Tom was a super sensitive child, and since early childhood his creative behavior and his own personal expectations had created frustration for him. His high intelligence in creative areas gave him far more desire to learn things than he was able to accomplish with his lower verbal abilities. This often results in the child feeling pressure not so much from the environment but from his own expectations. Then, when an adult also expresses a desire to see him do better there will be an intensification of the frustration. This is much like the situation where we do something we are displeased with followed by having someone else tell us how dumb we are for doing it. We all usually overreact to being caught in what we feel is something "dumb."

It is not that hemispheric difference is the problem so much as the consequences of that difference. With assistance and effort, particularly when the child does have adequate verbal abilities, the problem can usually be overcome. Tom's spatial-creative style of learning set him up to feel the most ease with a whole-word gestalt manner of learning to read. Yet, unaware of this, the teachers had continued to assist him in learning phonetics. Any testing that might have been done would have indicated that Tom had adequate intelligence and should have been able to learn phonetically. Only when the differences in Tom's various intellectual or developmental skills were realized would the teachers have known that he first needed whole-word approaches followed later by more phonetic activities. Tom also assumed that he should learn phonetics, and yet he had great difficulty. This eventually not only frustrated him but left him feeling "dumb" and eventually determined to avoid it all.

Sometimes even if the teachers are aware of a child's difficulties, inaccurate information can result in a disaster for the child. The teachers, in the next case, had conferred with each other over a two-year period and had the school psychometrist complete an evaluation. In spite of all of their effort, critical information had been missed. Based on what they knew they referred the child to be placed in a class for the mildly mentally handicapped. The child did not qualify, on the basis of a full-scale I.Q., but the school had decided to place her in the program anyhow. This case shows a dramatic situation in which a lack of understanding between the relationship of verbal and performance I.Q. and other behaviors of a child can create a misdiagnosis of the child's needs.

Case Study 5

Name: Ginny
Age: 8.4, Grade 1
Present Date: 4/22/81
School and Home Setting: Ginny is in a rural school which is organized around a traditional curriculum structure. It is a modern school with good facilities and the teaching staff is well qualified and experienced. Ginny lives with her natural parents and two sisters, one aged seven and the other nine. The family lives in a modest home and the father is a factory worker making an adequate income. The mother does not work and spends all of her time with the children. Economically the family would be considered in the lower middle socioeconomic classification.

Developmental history: Ginny talked late, at about fourteen months, but there was no particular concern by the parents. She seemed normal except for being somewhat small for her age. She was under constant pediatric care and the pediatrician felt there were no abnormalities. She repeated first grade due to a lack of adequate progress the first year. Due to her small size for her age and to her lack of progress, the school felt she was immature both physically and developmentally. Now, during her second year in first grade she is not doing much better.

Problem precipitating Referral: In April the parents were informed that Ginny needed to either be retained again or be referred for testing to determine why she was not progressing. The school personnel, during the case review, stated that she was developmentally delayed and inferred that she was mildly retarded. Further, the team asked the parents to see their pediatrician to determine if there was some sort of physiological problem preventing her from making adequate physical growth. The pediatrician became upset because the school inferred that there was a physical problem that he had not diagnosed and that she was possibly retarded. He referred her for developmental assessment.

WISC-R Scores:

Verbal:
    Information – 4
    Similarities – 7
    Math – 5
    Vocabulary – 6
    Comprehension – 6
    Digit Span – 10
Nonverbal:
    Picture completion – 10
    Picture Arrangement – 12
    Block Design – 16
    Object Assembly – 9
    Coding – 8
Verbal I.Q. score: 73
Performance I.Q. score: 106

PIAT:
  Reading recognition — 2.2
  Reading comprehension — 2.6
WRAT: 2.1
Berry Developmental Test: 7-5
Draw a Person: Elaborate and well developed

Ginny is a very active, verbal, and appealing child. She is alert and responded to directions during the evaluation very well. She gives the impression of a child who is very perceptive of the world about her and a child who certainly is not mentally retarded. Yet, as can be seen, her verbal abilities are well below average.

When looking at the language and nonverbal data it is apparent that Ginny is a child with some sort of language difficulty and yet average to above average nonverbal competencies. The data must be looked at carefully to get some picture of how Ginny is processing information. She is doing quite well on general spatial manipulative skills but very poorly on language tasks. She is able, apparently, to recall a sequence of verbal information, i.e. the digit span score, and not so well in fine motor copying tasks, i.e. the coding score. All of this does not seem to be enough to give us a good picture. At this point we might agree with the teachers.

If we look at the reading scores achieved, early second grade in April of the school year, we would not agree with the teachers that she needs to repeat first grade. In fact, these scores would indicate that by fall she would be ready for second grade. Why did the teachers feel she needed to repeat again? Here we have to remember that on a reading test such as the PIAT or WRAT we are seeing much visual recognition and a very short period of involvement. In the classroom Ginny may be working far below the 2.2 reading level achieved on the reading tests. In fact this is the case. What do the teachers see in the classroom?

In the classroom Ginny displays a very short attention span when working on reading or any seatwork task. At one point the teachers felt she might have a visual problem and as it turned out she did need corrective lenses. But the wearing of glasses did not increase her attention span. The mystery deepens. In any case Ginny did not do well in phonetics, and the teachers reported that she was only at about middle first grade in their structured phonetics program.

The mother had an interesting comment concerning reading. Ginny loved to read to her at home and seemed to love to read stories over and over. The mother was a sight reader and simply told Ginny the words she did not know. Ginny was reading books at home that were for second graders and she was working on one for third graders. The mother had gotten them from the library. As might be guessed the mother felt Ginny was doing very well. When she suggested that the teachers might not be taking the right approach there was a significant decrease in school-to-home communication. Add conflict to the mystery of Ginny.

To solve the mystery, as in the last case, one had to look beyond the classroom and enter a dark area of information and speculation. The dark area was one the school could not touch. . . genetics. One of the things that struck us during the evaluation was how small Ginny was and further how tiny her mother was. We had to ask. The mother was small and so was her mother and both had been developmentally slow in language and general development. To make it all more interesting the father was only slightly taller than the mother. The pediatrician reinforced that on both sides of this family there was a general tendency to be somewhat small and delayed in physical development. So much for the physical "abnormality."

More intriguing is the fact that Ginny is in a private gymnastics program and is somewhat of an expert in her age-group, having won several gymnastics events. She loves to dance and since her mother has a private dance studio Ginny has been exposed to both gymnastics and dance since she was a little girl. Further, Ginny is quite creative and enjoys a number of craft projects, which her mother also participates in.

At this point we began to see one of those children who displays good nonverbal and motoric development but has difficulty with language. In Figures 6 and 7 we see examples of Ginny's drawing of a person and her Berry Developmental test. We consider her delayed language development a serious problem, but since she has been held back in school this will become less of a problem.

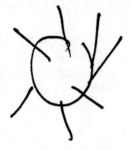

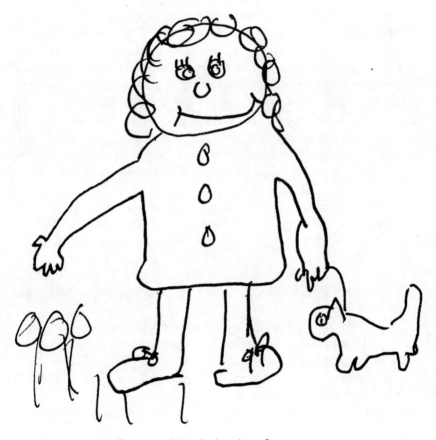

Figure 6. Ginny's drawing of a person.

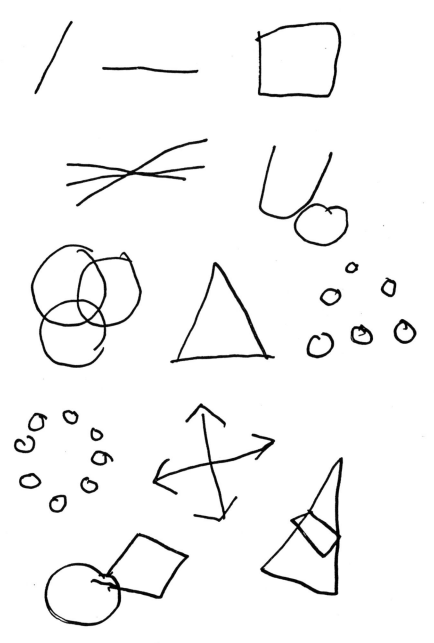

Figure 7. Ginny's Berry.

We tested Ginny's reading with a whole-word approach and found that when she is using this approach she is able to utilize context clues and very quickly master a few pages of reading at the late second grade level. Her phonetics skills are terrible, but when she is approached with a different method, whole to part, she can pick out prefixes and suffixes, word parts, compound words, and many other basic recognition units. Her spelling, as might be expected, is poorly done until rhythm and intonation are added and she then can recall quite well. It is obvious that a different approach in reading and spelling will soon make a difference. Following good progress some phonetic practice should be incorporated.

Ginny's case is not resolved so easily, however. As is the case in some school situations, the principal and the teachers were offended by both the intervention of the pediatrician and the outside assessment of her needs and were unwilling to change their program. The mother eventually had to enroll Ginny in a private school where she did go on to second grade and where the teachers were willing to change her curriculum approach. Ginny currently is completing the second grade and is doing quite well. A reassessment of her language skills showed that she is progressing, and our prediction is that eventually she will fall within the average range of verbal functioning.

We have been blessed with mostly fine school settings and cooperative teachers. But occasionally, as in Ginny's case we come across a school where cooperation is not forthcoming. It reinforces our concern that much of the technology available today in child development and learning is not reaching our schools. Now that we are entering the computer-based education era, we find a growing concern that the increasing difficulty, not only of understanding children but of utilization of new teaching methodologies, will be even less effective to help children like Ginny.

Ginny's case is an example of another problem we often see in educational philosophy. While recent years have shown that the concept of a fixed I.Q. is somewhat archaic, many educators still operate on the notion that whatever the intelligence level of the child may be it is unlikely to change. The problem is twofold; the average child or a child without any significant developmental problems does indeed maintain a somewhat steady level of intellectual functioning. Secondly, while the I.Q. test does not measure true intelligence, it is taken as a manifestation of intelligence by most educators. We assume that most children can benefit from increased stimulation, i.e. genetic factors and environment operate to maximize potential. In cases where there is a generalized competency with specific difficulties we work to maximize the child's capabilities and then work on skills. In a case such as Ginny's it was assumed that her overall communication competencies could be improved with learning and effort. We do not rely then, merely on the achieved I.Q. score as an indication of potential, rather, it is an indication of functional level. In cases of extreme differences in verbal and performance competencies, we work toward both understanding the differences in learning and behavior, and improving the deficit area. Sometimes we fail. In many children the gross differences in hemispheric function are unchangeable; then we have to teach the child differently, along with teaching him how to deal with his differences. But we always work to equalize the two modes of functioning to the greatest degree possible. This is not consistent with the philosophy that states that a child's intelligence is somewhat fixed. Such a notion dooms many children, like Ginny, to increasing incompetence. To have left Ginny with first graders or to have put her in a class with mentally retarded children would have most likely given her little stimulation and decreased the possibility of altering her potential.

There are many children for whom stimulation will not work due to a "pervasive" incompetence. It is the task of the educator and school psychologist to seek out those children where such a condition does not exist even though the test scores may seem to indicate this is so.

In the following case we have an example of what happens to a child when his I.Q. scores label him and subsequent expectations doom him to a world where he cannot succeed. This is a rather dramatic case but, unfortunately, it is not an exception.

Case Study 6

Name: Jerry
Age: 15-1

Present Date: 6/25/81

Jerry had just completed the eighth grade and was ready for high school. But he did not plan to go, at least he did not until the juvenile authorities picked him up just before school was out.

Home and School Setting: Jerry lives with his natural mother, one brother, and three sisters. Jerry is the second oldest of the children still living at home. The father does not live with the family but Jerry sees him quite often and helps him in his plumbing business. The parents live on a modest income and appear to care fairly well for the children. Jerry has two brothers who are grown and no longer live at home. Since the father left home some six years ago the mother has been the sole manager of the family and she finds it very difficult. Jerry attends a public school in a lower middle-class urban area.

Problem Precipitating the Referral: During the first and second semester, Jerry was warned several times about being truant from school. After repeated warnings and a lack of response, he was finally referred to the juvenile authorities. During the final weeks of school Jerry was picked up by the juvenile authorities and eventually ended up in the Juvenile Detention Center where a hearing was scheduled for late in June. Several contacts were made with the family prior to the actual detention and an assessment of Jerry's personality and general competence assessment had been completed. When he was finally picked up and detained a court lawyer referred him to the authors for an independent evaluation to be provided for the hearing.

Our own evaluation was completed prior to reviewing the court's records, which is our usual approach to avoid contamination of our own assessment. Upon reviewing the records concerning the court's evaluation and assessment, we were depressed. Before reviewing our own assessment, we will present a summary of the findings from the court.

Social Service Assessment: Without going into extensive discussion of the family interviews it should be of interest to summarize the social service assessment here.

> Jerry is a Caucasian male who is experiencing court referrals for school truancy. He has a pattern of school failure consistent with delinquency. Jerry's family has other siblings who have had similar

problems including drop-outs and school truants. Apparently the mother is not able to coerce or convince her children to go to school. At this point in time it appears somewhat bleak that Jerry will continue school while living at home because of his failure to achieve in the past. A foster home or institutional living arrangement may have to be sought.

Additional evaluations of speech, hearing, vision, and general perceptual motor function all fell within the normal range. An occupational assessment yielded a recommendation that Jerry would enjoy a job related to mechanical activities.

A psychological study had been completed approximately a year prior to Jerry's detainment. The following is a summary of the scores and the recommendations:

WISC–R Scores:

Verbal I.Q. Score – 77

Performance I.Q. Score – 135

Full Scale I.Q. Score – 103 Classification: Normal (Average)

PIAT:

Recognition – 3.8

Comprehension – 5.8

Spelling – 3.0

Also given were several psychological tests, including the Rorschach, Rotter Incomplete Sentences, Projective Drawings, and Thematic Apperception Test. We will summarize some of the statements made by the examiner.

1. Jerry has many underlying emotional and personal problems that have a depressing effect on his capacity to think in a logical manner.
2. The examinations reveal a verbally impoverished, intellectually depressed, nonverbal and inexpressive youngster.
3. Outwardly he can appear stubborn, negativistic, and he frequently manipulates others through procrastination, impressiveness, and unresponsiveness. His passive resistive behavior tends to predominate, and he remains evasive, uninvested, and he reveals a tendency to escape from situations that make him uncomfortable.
4. His environment is seen as threatening, fearful and unhappy. He is concerned with disapproval and feelings of acceptance

by others, and he maintains a discouraged, overwhelmed, and overpowering sense of futility and disappointment.

5. Jerry is a child of average intellectual functioning who reveals a fairly depressed level of intellectual and emotional performance.

6. Jerry needs to be placed in psychotherapy where a reassuring and protective adult can aid him in dealing with his anxiety and his sense of chronic depression that causes him to avoid painful situations.

It sounded as if Jerry was ready to be placed in a basket and carted off, unceremoniously, to the mental junk heap. This summary along with the social service information gave a most depressing picture of Jerry. It was fortunate we had not read all of this prior to seeing him.

Our own assessment was so dramatically different that it was obvious that the courts would have some trouble dealing with our findings.

WISC–R Scores:

Verbal:
Information — 5
Similarities — 5
Math — 4
Vocabulary — 7
Comprehension — 7
Digit Span — 7

Performance:
Picture Completion — 16
Picture Arrangement — 15
Block Design — 15
Object Assembly — 17
Coding — 12

Verbal I.Q. Score: 73
Performance I.Q. Score: 135

PIAT:
Recognition — 3.8
Comprehension — 5.1

WRAT: 3.4

Bender Gestalt: Excellent, above average
DAP: Excellent

This case requires several changes in our usual thinking about children and their behavior. The decision, prior to our involvement in the case, was to send Jerry to a closed reformatory for boys. It was one of those wonderfully archaic, red brick institutions where adolescents are placed for a year or so in order to be "reformed." It sounds like something impossible but in many states these institutions still detain boys who have no criminal records and further, no record of any sort of crime except running away or being truant. These boys are detained with other boys who are proven delinquents having criminal records. Many of those boys are chronic offenders with offenses including stealing cars and, would you believe, rape, and murder.

We saw Jerry on a sunny afternoon. He reflected that attitude, and though he was somewhat anxious he was positive and willing to cooperate. In essence, he seemed to be willing to do his best for he understood, from his lawyer, that we might be able to help him. Frankly, he was frightened about being in the detention center and even more fearful about being sent to the "reformatory." Jerry had never been away from home overnight until he was taken to the juvenile center. It was our impression that our results were valid and at this writing, nearly a year later, we were correct.

Jerry is a dramatic case of hemispheric difference. Due to the great difference we had to assume that genetic or early childhood deprivation were operating and had effectively delayed or retarded verbal development. According to our evaluation, Jerry was operating with a six-year difference between functional abilities in verbal and spatial-creative factors. One has difficulty looking into another's mind and imagining what the world would be like with that degree of difference between one's ability to create imagery mentally in nonverbal intelligence and to attempt to organize verbal information. Jerry was no more capable than a ten-year-old in verbal function and well over sixteen years old in the production of creative intelligence. One becomes somewhat defenseless in a verbal world with that sort of difference.

The confusion, frustration, anxiety, and outright fear that existed for Jerry were real, and any attempt to measure personality function, particularly with older tests designed for adults with psychological pathology, would have been devastatingly in error.

Our first concern was to attempt to determine Jerry's feelings and hopes relative to school and himself. What we found, through interviewing, was a boy with a very positive and immature self-concept. Teachers described him as a cooperative boy when he was in school and a boy who sought assistance from teachers. His one area of difficulty was in physical education where the teacher, even by his own admission, was abrasive and aggressive with Jerry. The teacher thought Jerry did not try hard enough, and said Jerry frequently did not dress because he forgot his gym clothes. We have had enough experience with preadolescent and adolescent boys to know that super-sensitive and shy boys often avoid the dressing room. Jerry, it turned out, was one of those boys. Remember, we are dealing with a boy who has the mental organization skills of a ten-year-old, living in a world of teenage boys. The teacher simply took the same aggressive approach he did with other boys and felt Jerry would "shape up." He did not. He ran instead, and there was no one who knew the problem or was in a position at the right time to find out.

But, as Jerry explained to us, there was another problem. In middle school, since fourth grade, he was placed in a class for the mentally retarded. He tried to explain that he was not dumb like those other kids. How did this boy, this gifted nonverbal boy, tell his teachers that? He could not prove it.

In frustration Jerry had taken to skipping school and not telling his mother. He had found some "friends" who also cut school and he began to hang out with them. Fortunately, Jerry was just beginning to relate to an out-group and was not yet part of the gang. He would rather go to school because he had promised his father he would.

The courts, as they have in so many other cases, accepted our findings and allowed Jerry and his mother to follow our recommendations. We have found that the courts do not really want to detain boys like Jerry, but they are reliant on the assessment they receive from professionals. In this case it was critical that the evaluation not only point to a logical basis for Jerry's behavior but also show some reasonable plan whereby he could remain in school and make it to class. This was accomplished with little difficulty once a more realistic picture was gained of his needs.

The first overall picture we must form of Jerry is that of a highly creative, sensitive, and spatially oriented boy. This carries with it, particularly with the significantly high creative ability, an intuitiveness about others through his ability to read nonverbal communication. The question becomes, in what emotional direction does this sensitivity move, toward hostility and defensiveness or toward acceptance and positiveness? An individual who is highly sensitive to personal feelings and those of other people must in some manner react to those feelings. In Jerry we found, both from his school record and reports from the mother, a consistent story. Jerry was a somewhat shy boy who generally tended to be friendly and cooperative. This had been true throughout his regular and special education experience. We did not see an overly sensitive boy who was defensive and hostile. This added to our belief that the psychological tests were measuring situational factors of the test situation, which he did not have the verbal abilities to evaluate, and consequently he responded with anxiety and fear. Further, due to his highly creative orientation it is unlikely that he could have verbalized or organized a successful understanding of the test situation.

Jerry tended to be creative in his drawings, and his interpretation of designs or ink blots would have reflected a combination of creative interpretation and the underlying anxiety of the test situation. Our conclusion was that the depressive and anxious pathology that the examiner was seeing came from an unsuspected source, the situation and the examiner's manner rather than from Jerry. The examiner, it appears, was unable to understand the creative mind and unable to reflect compassion for the subject. . . Jerry. Had these two factors been present Jerry would most likely have presented himself differently. This is one reason that projective tests, based on both pathological perimeters and examiner bias, tend to· occasionally display what the test seeks to find, pathology.

Jerry's drawing of a person in Figure 8, demonstrates not only a creative mind but also some skill in drawing which is consistent with our findings in general cerebral competencies. There could be some interpretation of the fact that the individual is running. We could ask what he is running from? Or we could accept it for what it is, the expression of some inner imagery of the moment, reflecting more of the child's potential than reflecting some pathological response. We chose the former. The drawing also displays an interesting factor of hemisphericity. Left-handed, or right hemispherically oriented individuals, often draw figures from the side view with the face pointing to the right, while right-handed individuals most often face them to the left. Jerry's drawing is consistent with his high right hemispheric orientation.

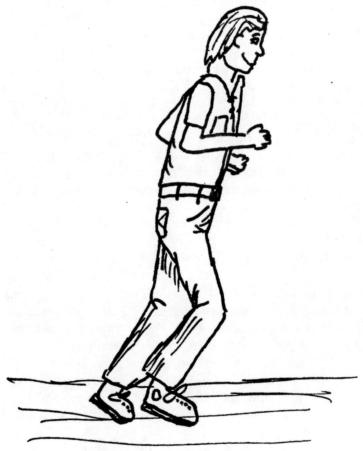

Figure 8. Jerry's drawing of a person.

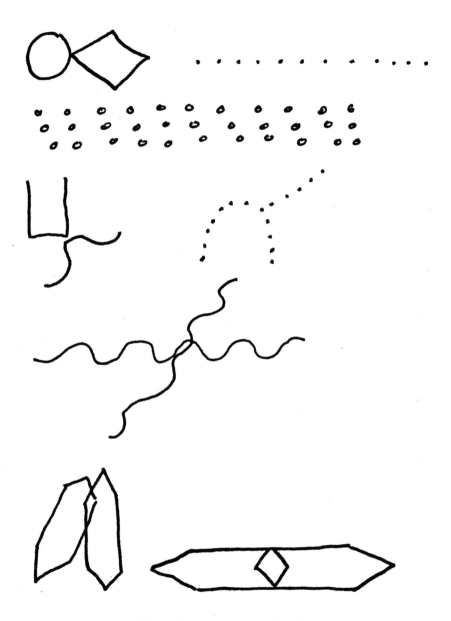

Figure 9. Jerry's Bender Gestalt.

Jerry's rendering of the Bender Gestalt seen in Figure 9, while demonstrating some minor motoric difficulties, is fairly well organized and absent from serious emotional indicators. There is no significant pathology here either.

Our problem then, was to ascertain what overall approaches should be initiated to assist Jerry in attending school and continuing to develop a positive self-image and academic skills. His reading turned out to be similar to that found in the original assessment. His writing skills were adequate though, and as might be expected, spelling was a disaster. Reading would have to be included in the program as would much assistance in verbal learning. There was obvious competency in spatial and mechanical skills which could result in an effective vocational program. Our recommendation placed Jerry in the learning disabled category with serious verbal and language function difficulties.

Jerry would need to be in the slow track in regular coursework but not in a class for mentally retarded. His work would have to be modified and he would need resource teacher assistance with some coursework being taken in a learning disabilities resource room. He would need to be programmed into vocational education with resource assistance for both Jerry and the teachers. He would need weekly counseling, for improved self-concept and continued school attendance, by someone who could show a real interest in him and form a relationship upon which Jerry could rely.

All of these recommendations were available within the high school that he would attend in the fall. The original examiners had not known the nature or the availability of school programming and therefore could not have foreseen how Jerry might have been helped. Theirs was strictly an evaluation of the child before them. In our work we find that knowing the available resources is as critical as making some sort of diagnosis. Further, the professional has to know something of the state and federal laws pertaining to the handicapped, and the needed information to give the school personnel so that they can make a judgement of their resources and the child's needs. For Jerry, in all of this, there would be priorities if we were to get him involved and motivated toward school attendance. It would not be enough to rely on his fear of going to a reform school to get him to attend school. We

had to create an atmosphere of trust and present options that would interest him and take advantage of positive intrinsic motivation, not external threats and a desire to avoid punishment.
The following priorities were established:

1. Jerry and his mother would first have to go to the school to meet the special education personnel in learning disabilities, and be assured that he would not have to attend classes for the mentally retarded.
2. Secondly Jerry would have to participate in a case conference in which his options would be outlined in a positive way. He would have to be taken to the vocational program to meet some of the teachers and see what those options meant in concrete form.
3. Finally, Jerry would have to meet and be counseled by the resource teacher who would become his advocate in the school program. His program and schedule would have to be constructed to provide as little confusion as possible for Jerry. He would need to come to school for summer work to prepare for the fall. He would, at that time, familiarize himself with the environment and the nature of his schedule. During the summer session he would receive individual assistance in reading, and study skills, along with developing a feeling of security and trust in the school personnel.

All of this was tentatively approved with one phone call to a resource teacher in the secondary program. Jerry would not go to reform school, but he would learn to accept responsibility and perhaps, for the first time, begin to feel that someone not only cared, but understood his needs and his capabilities.

This all required much effort on the part of the school personnel, but the program was set up with a minimum of difficulty. In the fall Jerry went to high school. At this writing, nearly a year later, Jerry is doing well. There have been problems, and on a few occasions he did not make it to school. But, with the strength of a probation program and the positive approach of the school, absences were minimal and the courts and the school cooperated to solve what could have been a very difficult problem. If Jerry had gone to reform school he would now be sixteen, on the streets, and learning skills in delinquency.

This case is not unusual but it points up again how critical the relationship and interdisciplinary communication between the schools and the courts or other community agencies is, if we are to assist boys like Jerry. Finally, it was the general concepts of hemisphericity that made it possible to see Jerry's needs in a productive way. It was not that Jerry was "right brained" or only that he was a highly creative boy with poor language, it was the integration of the notions of hemisphericity with other data that assisted in achievement of success for Jerry. This case illustrates how such concepts may begin to change our notion about personality testing and the older theories of pathology. Without the concepts of child development and hemisphericity, Jerry would have been lost both to society and to himself.

Chapter 5

CASE STUDIES — GROUP C

THESE last case studies include two longitudinal views of children and how they grew. In the hundreds of high spatial children we have seen over the years many have now grown into adolescence and beyond. For the most part it has been a loving and pleasing experience. But it has often been a frustrating and uncertain experience too, for in the process of being an advocate for children, one often finds himself between the establishment and the children. Sometimes the establishment is a teacher, sometimes a principal and a whole diagnostic team, and sometimes it is the parent. From initial diagnosis to the first crisis, when the suggestions you make do not seem to be working, the child may be involved with the law or end up in juvenile court. We have rescued children from juvenile centers, from mental institutions, drug centers, from angry school personnel, and from themselves. Never was the feeling one of self-confidence and satisfaction at having beaten the system, but always it has been with some sorrow that the child had to be saved at all. Most of these children should never have to be saved. In the end, when the curtain falls and the players and the audience have gone home, you are left realizing that if you had expected a special thanks you would be disappointed. Working with children and doing whatever it is that professionals in child development and care are supposed to do, is a career, it is not a play in which the director is applauded. In real life one does what he can and expects that any thanks that come must come from intrinsic satisfaction. These cases illustrate, over the time of their development, the sorts of problems that confront these children who have special creative abilities. In the end one comes to appreciate them and to feel privileged to have played a part in a worthwhile human drama. It is nice to find special needs that exist in a child and relate them to teachers and other professionals where the story is continued without your knowledge. But it is a challenge and an opportunity to truly help children when you can grow up with them, year by year, and not only suffer as they suffer, but also know the joy they feel when at last they believe in themselves.

Case Study 7

Name: Billy
Age at first contact: 4-8
Date: 2/15/74
Age at last contact: 12-10
Date: 4/15/82

Billy first came to the clinic when he was four years old. The parents at that time were concerned about his maturity and readiness to begin kindergarten the next fall. If he was immature, it was their hope that some sort of assistance might be given so that he could be ready for school. Both parents were college graduates and the mother did not work outside the home. They lived in a middle class suburban area where the schools were some of the best in the area. The parents were conscientious and were quite concerned about the education of their children. One got the impression that this was a typical, well-adjusted family and that relative to parenting skills, this couple would probably exemplify the modern young couple. We were right in that assumption but our "career" with Billy had not begun.

Developmental history: Billy had been a difficult child from the onset. He was a fussy and active boy who tried his parents' patience. He had tantrums at a young age, cried often, and was quite difficult to hold. He had been adopted at five months of age from a foster home. It was believed that he had not received much affection in the foster home and there was concern that some abuse had occurred. He displayed normal language and motor development, with no significant difficulties noted until he entered preschool at the age of four. In preschool Billy exhibited a high activity level, resistance to teacher instruction, unwillingness to participate in games other than those he chose, and a great deal of emotional variability. At the beginning of the second semester the teacher informed the parents of these problems, and the fact that Billy's fine motor skills were not developing as well as they should.

Precipitating event: Billy displayed an overly active behavioral pattern, poor organization both in behavior and fine motor skills, and a tendency to resist teacher direction and group socialization skills.

Data obtained at age 4-6:
WIPPSI Scores:

Verbal:
　　Information – 15
　　Vocabulary – 13
　　Arithmetic – 10
　　Similarities – 10
　　Comprehension – 19
Performance:
　　Animal house – 10
　　Picture Completion – 15
　　Mazes – 14
　　Geometric design – 13
　　Block Design – 15
Verbal I.Q. Score: 121
Performance I.Q. Score: 123
Peabody Picture Vocabulary: 120
Draw A Person: Adequate
Geometric Design: Above average
Letter recognition: None

Behavioral factors: At this time Billy was demonstrating many demanding behaviors at home. He was resistive to discipline and tended to have tantrums if he could not do what he wanted to do. In his preschool he tended to dominate other children and take toys away from them. This information caused the parents to become concerned that he might be too immature for kindergarten the next fall.

　　Billy was seen as a boy who resisted drawing and fine motor skills though there were no significant problems in this area. He did not like to participate in teacher-directed activities and sub-sequently had not learned many of the listening skills, to attend to and follow directions, and other important preschool skills. Both the teacher and the parents did not feel he would be ready for kindergarten in the fall.

Billy's situation is very common. Parents and teachers often see such behavioral patterns as representing immaturity, but most often immaturity is much more complex than the skill of listening to and following directions. Some children are unable to do this because of general immaturity. Yet, it must be decided if such behaviors are the result of an inability to attend or if, as in Billy's case, the child is "out of bounds" and is avoiding following directions.

As can be seen in Billy's case, there are adequate verbal and nonverbal abilities to organize attention, to learn needed skills, and to adapt to a preschool setting. His difficulties were not from immaturity, but rather from a developmental difference, i.e., he is able to learn but is deterministic, egocentered, and unwilling to accept authority and direction. This is very different than immaturity and if he is retained with younger children next year he will not "grow out of it." He must be assisted in "learning his way out of it." Immaturity is one of the most common reasons for retaining young children in preschool and it is often a mistake. Instead of additional time, they often need increased structure and direction.

While Billy received an above average score on the geometric designs on the WIPPSI, as shown in Figure 10, at this age only a slight advantage can give the impression of excellent skills, when in fact they are not all that exceptional. In the drawing of a triangle he demonstrated difficulty in angulation and in making the diagonal lines. This is also illustrated in the triangle which, though passable, is not well done. Even the circle displays a great deal of inaccuracy. Billy's drawing of a person was adequate as can be seen in Figure 11.

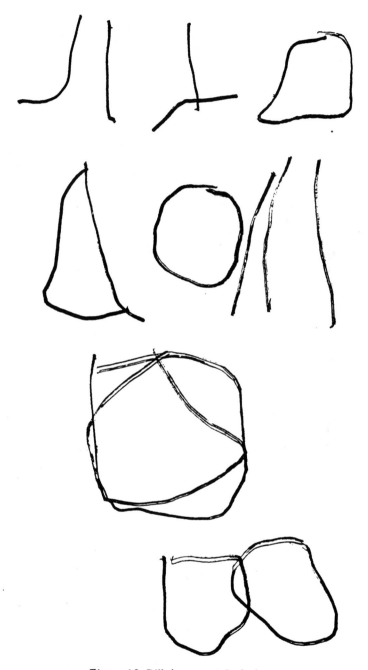

Figure 10. Billy's geometric designs.

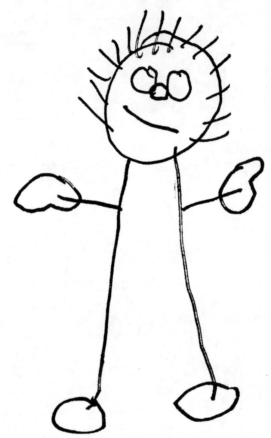

Figure 11. Billy's drawing of a person.

Based on the evidence it was recommended that Billy attend an all-day kindergarten the next fall so that he would experience an increased level of stimulation, and an increased amount of time required on task. For boys like Billy, who are active and alert, it is often desirable to increase the normal half-day experience to a full day, so that more time can be given to assisting them.

Second Contact one year later: Age: 5-6
WISC–R Scores:

Verbal:
  Information – 10

Similarities – 12
Arithmetic – 13
Vocabulary – 14
Comprehension – 12
Digit Span – 9
Performance:
    Picture completion – 13
    Picture arrangement – 15
    Block design – 15
    Object Assembly – 16
    Coding – 9
Verbal I.Q. Score: 99
Performance I.Q. Score: 125
PIAT:
    Recognition – 1.4
    Comprehension – 1.4
WRAT: 1.5
Berry Developmental: Above average.

This evaluation was completed as Billy was finishing his first year in a full-day private kindergarten. The school was highly structured and the teachers used much behavioral modification with him. The results are obvious. His fine motor skills have increased significantly, he has gone from no letter recognition to early first grade level work in reading, and the parents reported a decrease in resistive behavior at home.

But some interesting changes occurred that raised many questions from the parents. His verbal I.Q. had dropped over twenty points while his nonverbal intelligence had remained essentially the same. Why? The first factor is that there was a change in the specific tests used. We gave the WIPPSI the first year and switched to the WISC for the second testing. There is a great deal of difference between the two tests, and though one cannot really account totally for the I.Q. difference on that basis, the two tests do require quite different levels of performance and organization. We speculated that, in fact, there was an actual decrease in the rate of language development during the year as more overall organization was required of Billy. This plateauing effect is sometimes seen in young children when they must integrate developmental abilities in some way. Overall development may improve while specific areas may appear to decline. It is not that Billy's verbal abilities declined so much as there was a change in overall integration, a basic difference in the two tests, and the variability of examiner error and method of giving the tests. The two tests were given by different examiners. Our overall experience though suggested that there had been some decline in language development rate and, along with the other factors, we were seeing a slightly depressed language score relative to potential.

As can be seen in Figures 12 and 13, Billy's drawing skills had improved significantly, showing a gain of much more than a year. This supported the high spatial skill development over verbal growth as seen in the second testing.

The kindergarten teacher was asked to complete the Devereux Elementary Rating Scale, which is a survey designed to measure the child's behavioral adjustment in school. The teacher felt that Billy was pretty much within the normal range in general behavioral and social skills. The Devereux is published by the Devereux Foundation in Devon, Pennsylvania.

Things were looking pretty good at the end of kindergarten. We had a child who seemed to be integrating his abilities pretty well. We did not see Billy for some years, until the parents called to have him reevaluated due to behavioral difficulties at school.

(*Third contact:*)
Age: 10-6, 5th grade
WISC–R Scores:
Verbal:
    Information – 13
    Similarities – 9
    Arithmetic – 10
    Vocabulary – 12
    Comprehension – 12
    Digit Span – 10
Performance:
    Picture Completion – 11
    Picture Arrangement – 14

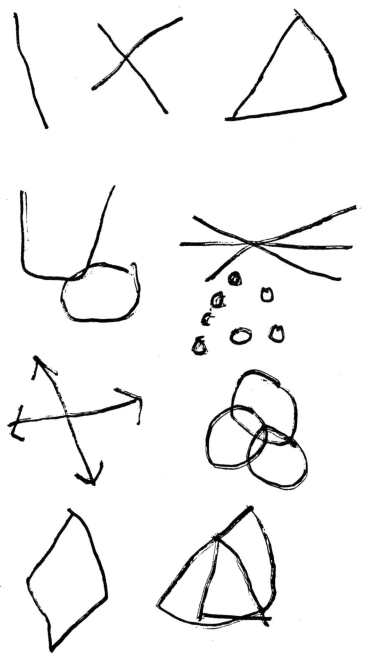

Figure 12. Billy's kindergarten drawing.

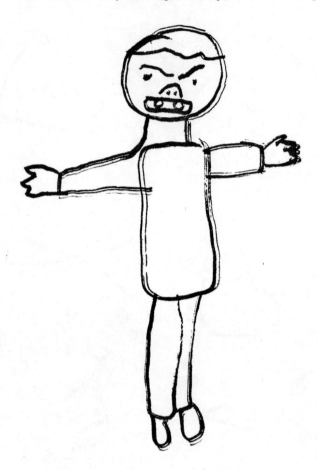

Figure 13. Billy's kindergarten drawing.

Block Design – 14
Object Assembly – 16
Coding – 12
Verbal I.Q. Score: 107
Performance I.Q. Score: 124
PIAT:
    Recognition – 6.1
    Comprehension – 6.8

WRAT:
   Recognition – 5.9
   Spelling – 3.8
   Math – 6.2
Berry Developmental: 12-0
Draw a Person: Creative

It sounded like an old story, revived. In the interim of years since we had seen Billy, he continued to progress through school. But he also retained many of the behavior problems that surfaced in preschool but which seemed to subside following kindergarten. They had not. Apparently the excellent programming and behavioral modification in kindergarten had been effective in containing his impulsivity and poor social skills. But while kindergarten had been a good year for Billy, as he continued in school, the absence of a continuous program of behavioral management had resulted in poor behavioral skills.

The parents had contacted a local child guidance clinic for therapy during his second and third grade years and this had helped somewhat. But at the present he was getting into fights at school, was resistive to directions, and was generally not doing well. There were also continuing problems at home with lying (or fabrication as we called it), some minor stealing, and abusive behavior with a younger sister who was three years younger than Billy.

We administered the CPQ, Children's Personality Questionnaire, to Billy. The CPQ is a well-constructed questionnaire that gives a readout of a child's general personality characteristics. We felt there was a need for additional information about his general personality. That test yielded the following information.

Billy was found to be a very reserved and verbally capable boy. He displayed adequate emotional stability, although he was somewhat excitable and demanding. He was not overly assertive but was not passive either. He was pretty typical in aggressiveness, and his general surgency (overall mental attitude) was average. He was though, quite expedient, and tended to structure rules to fit himself rather than those of authorities. He was somewhat shy and quite circumspect about himself and probably had some concerns that he was not expressing. He tended to be somewhat impulsive and displayed some degree of psychological stress.

His overall psychological profile tended to suggest a boy who was not in serious emotional difficulty but was probably an opportunist and manipulative. There was much egocentricity and a need to be recognized and loved.

Billy's mother was a tall, aggressive, and demanding woman who liked to have control. She tended to intellectualize emotions and was not a very affectionate woman, though she tried to program this as well as she understood it. The father was a nonaggressive, kind, and quiet male who was dominated by the mother. He also tried to intellectualize love and parenting and did so successfully, except he had problems with conflict and confrontation. Both parents were socially conscious and the problems with Billy at school were very painful for them. There is little doubt that they tried to talk Billy out of his problems and had difficulty showing affection. They often became frustrated with Billy; and without "honest" affection, he most likely engaged them in a game of guess and run, with no real resolution in the parent-child conflicts.

Billy was also exhibiting very consistent verbal and performance abilities relative to our testing several years before. Apparently we were correct in assuming that the earlier verbal and performance abilities were representative of his actual competencies. This meant that we did have a child with highly efficient creative abilities; and while his verbal abilities were adequate, without constant love and structure, he would tend to avoid verbal tasks and constrictions on his behavior.

In this case we had a combination of important variables that were somewhat predictable over time and which were borne out in Billy's development. The following factors were important in this case:

1. Poor early attachment and bonding, which can produce a nonaffectual child.

2. Creative abilities and higher spatial skills causing a tendency toward nonverbal function. This results in some cases in impulsive and sensitive behavior, fantasy, a tendency to fabricate, to avoid responsibility, and a highly active and

ego-centered personality. In Billy's case the added poor emotional bonding would have intensified his asocial behavior and poor peer adjustment.

3. Reading skills were initially poor but, as we found, he used a highly spatial approach in reading combined with some phonetics, and was able to do well in reading. He tended to have difficulty on tests requiring specific facts, but he was able to compensate through overall awareness and recall of information.

4. He displayed a lack of good value orientation and a tendency toward being an opportunist in school and social relationships.

5. Billy needed much affection, recognition, structure, and parental and school limit setting. He also needed socially acceptable outlets for his active behavior.

6. The parents needed counseling for their own disappointment in Billy and perhaps assistance in learning how to accept him and communicate real affection. The parents had to recognize their own inability to accept Billy and their tendency to hold in their anger and express it through rejection and denial.

There are many aspects to this case that would excite psychologists and have them asking for more. But in a "nutshell" there were three major factors that needed to be focused on in Billy's case. Billy had poor early attachment and distrust for adults and yet had a highly creative mind which gave a basis for much interest in affection. Secondly, Billy was blessed, or not so blessed, with parents who could not give him basic affection and tended to intellectualize, instead of working within Billy's style of highly active and creative interaction. The parents had not reinforced the sports, active outdoor play, and interests that would have given Billy expression for his abilities. Thirdly, Billy had continuously slipped through the cracks of instruction at school, and though he had problems, he was never "bad" enough to warrant any special attention. Therefore, each year, an unaware teacher missed his need for affection and high structure. Things just drifted along year after year with nothing ever being really resolved. Things had not gotten tremendously worse, but the stage was set, here in preadolescence, for a deepening of Billy's difficulty.

With these sorts of children, when they enter adolescence, with all of the attendant problems of self-identity and an increased need for affection and acceptance, they are vulnerable to several negative experiences. Here finally, they will have to resolve their own self-concept structure or enter adulthood with a tendency toward sociopathic behavior. This implies that they will attempt to continue to manipulate others without a sense of inner competency. They may tend to experiment with drugs due to their high spatial and sensory orientation. They may seek out peers who also have adjustment problems and begin to rebel against authority, since rebellion has been lurking, unresolved, throughout childhood. Difficulties in school adjustment, poor academic competencies, difficulties with peers, and a lack of solid home management all lay the basis for potential delinquency in adolescence. Billy, for all of his economic advantages, had all of the criteria for a real behavioral rebellion in adolescence. We were not so concerned about his present behavior as the future potentials which existed.

At this point it was important to initiate an overall program of assistance for Billy and the school, which would be ongoing into the next year. We are not convinced, after years of work in therapy situations in both institutions and the community, that boys like Billy benefit from conventional counseling. First, boys like Billy have to be dealt with in activity situations, and the influence of adults has to pervade their world everyday and not just during weekly family counseling situations. Secondly, it was unlikely that the parents would make any real change in their behavior in that their intellectualization and defenses were problems in themselves which could take many hours of work. Billy did not have time to wait until his parents could get their difficulties resolved. Further, their behavior and adaptive skills worked fine in their social and work world. Finally, Billy needed a special person with whom he could identify and who could organize his general behaviors in productive ways. In light of all of this, the following recommendations were made and the program was carried out for more than two years on a variable contact basis:

1. Billy was assigned to a counselor who was a male teacher in a different school. This individual was very athletic and was to engage Billy in the development of athletic skills, particularly football, which he liked very much. He also liked wrestling and his counselor was a wrestler in college. The counselor would meet with Billy once a week for the remainder of the school year and continue as long as the relationship seemed productive. The counselor would encourage the parents to engage Billy in other activities in the community.

2. The parents would attend weekly counseling for the purpose of establishing behavioral management techniques until they felt capable and comfortable with the skills. This would then be discontinued with infrequent sessions when the parents felt such assistance was needed.

3. The counselor and one of our staff would meet with the teachers at school on a monthly basis to assist in providing effective behavioral management there. Billy would be put on behavioral contracts and given assistance in following through with appropriate rewards.

4. Specific classroom instructions included assistance in developing study skills, planned and consistent study times at home and school, and alteration of some assignments to allow Billy to take tests on a verbal basis. He was enrolled in a special creative writing program during the summer, and in the fall additional time was given in assisting him in this area. The school was given instructions to intervene in situations where negative peer contacts seemed to be developing.

Billy, at this writing, is on the school wrestling team and the contacts with the special counselor, which lasted over a year, are no longer needed. The program has worked well. But the parents have been instructed to come for six-month reevaluations through Billy's high school years to assure that they manage his behavior well and that problems do not develop before teachers and school personnel are alert to his needs.

Case Study 8

Name: Max

Date: 6/78
Age at second contact: 14-10
Age at third contact: 15-10
Age at last contact: 16-2
Initial Contact: Age, 13-5, seventh grade

Max was a handsome boy. In our records, as we sometimes do to assist ourselves in recalling a child, we noted that he looked like a young Victor Mature. That received mixed reviews from the staff, most of whom had never heard of Victor Mature. That tends to make one feel old. In any case, Max was a muscular and athletic boy of thirteen years who smiled easily and was quite cooperative. The parents were both physicians and had one other child who was a girl, two years younger than Max. The parents were quite involved in their practice and both were quite naive about children, in fact, they were true intellectuals and dedicated to their profession. They admitted that they had not particularly planned on having children but were quite pleased when they discovered the wife was pregnant. We all wondered later if they really understood how it had all come about. In any case, they were very open and yet quiet people who seemed awed at their own parenthood.

Max had difficulty learning from the onset of school but the parents had always taken this in stride and still loved him in their own quiet and unassuming manner. In the seventh grade though, Max had significant problems keeping up in school, and the parents were called in and told that he was in need of some sort of special assistance. The school recommended that they get a tutor and that they have more frequent contacts with the school. The school did not, nor had they ever, recommended that any special testing be completed on Max. He was always a quiet and cooperative boy who smiled easily, but he never did very well in school. Everyone seemed to feel that he was simply immature and that next year he would "get it all together." He never did. *Developmental History*: Max displayed no significant difficulties as a young child. Although he had always been recognized as being somewhat immature, no one had ever been alarmed. He appeared to do his best, and fortunately it seemed to be enough to keep him moving along in school. There had been no special problems ever noted in his development. It was apparent, though, that his parents probably had never really paid that much attention to him. He liked to play alone, build things, and was able to manage on his own throughout much of his childhood. He had a good imagination and liked sports.

Precipitating event: At the end of the seventh grade the parents were advised that he should repeat that grade. There had been several school conferences with the parents during the year pointing out his problems. Though we were never told, it appeared that Max had been placed in a slow track when he started seventh grade, but the parents did not seem to truly grasp this concept. They were more concerned about his having to repeat seventh grade and brought him to find out, as they stated, why he had difficulty with reading comprehension, studying, and adapting to school. It seemed implausible, as will be seen, that these two parents could have been so oblivious to their own child's developmental differences for so long. We eventually accepted though, that these parents really did not understand the problem. They truly were two souls, committed to medical matters, who completely missed how a child might be slow. They were probably so involved in their own world that they assumed others thought as they did. It was an unusual experience to talk to them. It was like talking to two children about matters completely new to them. They were awed with each bit of information and were quite open to almost anything we said and would then ask, "How do we treat it?"

WISC–R Scores:

Verbal:

    Information – 6

    Similarities – 6

    Arithmetic – 7

    Vocabulary – 8

    Comprehension – 8

    Digit Span – 8

Performance:

    Picture Completion – 9

    Picture Arrangement – 14

Block Design — 13
Object Assembly — 13
Coding — 12
Verbal I.Q. Score: 81
Performance I.Q. Score: 115
PIAT:
Recognition — 6.8
Comprehension — 4.1
WRAT: 5.8
Berry Developmental: 14-10
Draw a Person: Immature

Max was very cooperative during the testing. The findings were somewhat surprising to us too. Max seemed to be an alert boy when talking to him and yet, once his verbal abilities had been revealed, his smiling and cooperative manner reinforced the fact that he was quite slow in verbal development. His verbal score of 81 was only a few points above that of the mildly mentally handicapped. Yet, his spatial creative intelligence was in the low-bright range. Max had been in good schools and they had worked hard with him. He read very much by a whole-word process with minimal use of phonetics. But he read pretty well considering his verbal abilities. Yet, there was little comprehension, and as can be seen on the reading scores, his comprehension was well below his recognition skills. He had learned the words but his verbal system failed him and he could not respond. In order to assist him in comprehension much language development would have to be done and it was not likely to have a significant impact at this age. He needed much assistance in the classroom and special assistance in a program for slow learners would be appropriate.

When Max's world was viewed from a realistic standpoint, it made more sense. He had difficulties in verbal comprehension but could compensate in social settings with the higher spatial intelligence. After all, much of communication is not verbal and Max could read people's behavior well. He was, as we mentioned, a quiet and unassuming child, and therefore there was no aggressiveness toward achievement. He loved his stereo, and building things at home, so his world was pretty much as he liked it. There was no need to struggle. He had few friends but this did not seem to bother him. He played baseball in the summer and liked tennis, which he played frequently. On the tennis court he looked like a handsome and capable youngster. He had only done one thing that had alarmed his father. He had smoked marijuana. That interested his father and he spent some time talking to Max about it. Max said he did not know where he got it, but he did not try to deny he had smoked it. He had smoked it at home apparently, and not with other boys.

All of this was explained to the parents who asked many unemotional questions and seemed intent on doing whatever was needed. Their reaction seemed curious to us. Many parents would have been both crushed and confused at the news that their child was nearly mentally retarded relative to school achievement.

It was recommended that the parents obtain a tutor for Max and that in the fall they should place him in a small private school where he would be more closely supervised by the teachers and where his peer associations could be monitored more easily. The school he had been attending was one of those super middle schools with more than a thousand students. Since the parents could afford a smaller school where some special assistance would be available, it was recommended that they place him there. In the past we had had a great deal of good experience with the school and felt that they could give him the needed attention.

Second contact: October, eighth grade
Age: 14-10

Max entered the private school and had done quite well. Everything seemed to be working as we had hoped. We heard from the parents in late October and the father was extremely distressed. Max was scheduled for a court hearing at the Juvenile Center following a complaint by a neighbor who stated that he had given her fourteen-year-old daughter "pot" to smoke and then asked her to engage in sexual behavior at his house. Needless to say the neighborhood became quite excited about this incident that the girl had reported to her parents. Before it all subsided, Max was painted as a delinquent who was on the road to becoming a rapist. Max was somewhat bewildered and embarrassed by it all and yet honest about what he had done. It was later discovered that the girl had supplied the "pot," and with some effort on our part, the case was dismissed with the recommendation that our office would provide counseling for Max. We knew that counseling would have little effect on a boy with a mental age of about ten to eleven years. He did not have any more incidents, however. The school did provide him with a good educational program and the year in the eighth grade ended successfully.

The next fall Max entered a local high school for ninth grade. The parents did not contact us at that time and so Max, along with his parents, made out a schedule for his high school program. The school did not have Max's records at that time and entered him in the regular school curriculum in a non-college preparation program.

Third Contact: Age, 15-10, ninth grade

In October the father called in somewhat of a panic. There was to be a conference with the parents, Max, and all of Max's teachers, due to his poor grades and his lack of willingness to cooperate in school. The father wanted us to attend the conference, which we agreed to do. Until we arrived at the meeting and spent some time listening to the teachers, we did not know that Max was not receiving any special assistance and was in all regular classes. It seemed impossible that he could have been programmed into regular classes without some assistance, but Max was not only in regular classes including algebra, and regular English, but neither the teachers nor the counselor conducting the meeting appeared to know anything about Max.

Max was, of course, in the meeting and the teachers, each in turn, told how he did not try in class, how he often just smiled instead of answering, how he didn't turn in his homework, and generally was a nonparticipant. The worst indictment seemed to be his seemingly uninterested and unconcerned attitude.

We sat in horror as a group of teachers assailed a boy who could not really understand what they were saying. He looked concerned and bewildered. He could read the anger and disgust on their faces. Following the teacher's comments the counselor in charge of the meeting asked us if we would like to give some information that might help the situation. By that time we were in shock; further, we did not want to have to say in front of Max, that he was, for all practical purposes, a mildly mentally handicapped boy who could not understand nor deal with their demands. We presented some history and softly suggested that Max had many learning difficulties. We asked the counselor if he had read any of the material which, by that time, had reached the school and was in Max's folder. The counselor said he had not really had time to look at it. We suggested that the meeting be adjourned with he and the parents meeting later after the information had been reviewed. The parents went home with Max and we went to the counselor's office.

The counselor obtained Max's folder and we reviewed the information with him. He was somewhat aghast at the record and was surprised that Max had been enrolled in regular classes. It had all been a mistake. We asked what could be done and he stated that in order to get special help Max would have to be tested by the school psychometrist.

We asked when the testing could be scheduled, and we were informed that it could take several weeks, but that he would try to speed up the process. The high school was a large school with more than 1,800 students. Apparently, Max could get lost in the shuffle. But there was nothing that could be done until the testing was completed.

In the next three weeks Max began to skip school and simply stayed home. He did not wander in the neighborhood or get into trouble. He did not understand what was happening and to avoid it all he simply stayed home. This resulted in several phone calls to the parents ending with a threat to call in juvenile authorities if he was not back in school at once. When the parents called we contacted the counselor who, unfortunately, had not been involved in the truancy problem and was unaware of it. In any case, he explained that Max's truancy problem was separate from the testing and he would have to return to school. We tried to explain that Max was drowning in mistakes, misunderstandings, and was in essence being forced out of school. It did not matter.

The testing was scheduled twice and Max missed one session and the psychometrist the other – 0 for Max and 0 for the school. We were now into December and Max was continuing to have worse problems in school. Finally the testing was accomplished and Max's schedule was changed. He was placed in a slow track and two vocational classes but he would have to take failing grades for most of what he had done the first semester.

Following Christmas vacation Max was doing better in the new program, but he was so far behind in the vocational classes that the teachers were somewhat irritated that he had been allowed to be entered with so little of the semester left. There were several disagreements between the vocational teachers and the counselor, and the counselor admitted that they were doing little to assist Max. The counselor stated that many of the vocational teachers resented the slow learners being placed in their classes. As might be expected, being caught in the middle, Max took his own route out and again missed school several times. He turned sixteen before the beginning of the second semester and the school excluded him, following a review of his attendance record and for "obvious" encouragability, for the remainder of the semester. Max was not angry, he simply gave up.

Last Contact: Age 16-2

We appealed the decision and a hearing was granted to the parents for the next month, which was March. The appeal hearing was finished before it began. The Dean of Boys presented Max's record and Max was allowed to talk. He said he wanted to go to school but did not know what to do. He was bewildered and nothing could have been more depressing than to watch a boy who could not defend himself, and parents who were shocked, run headlong into school regulations, school's rights, and other damaging and rigid rules that made it clear Max was an offending party. The Dean concluded his presentation in a coldly factual and legal manner stating that in that Max was now sixteen he was no longer legally entitled to school services due to his lack of willingness to attend school.

So, on a sunny day in early March Max left school for good. He did not know for sure why and his parents had given up. We saw Max at a local fast-food restaurant the following summer and he was cheerful as always. He told us he was working for a florist but did not make much money. We asked that he come to the office so that maybe we could help him get into night school. He said that he did not think he wanted to go back to school just yet.

At this writing we do not know what has happened to Max. There are a lot of Maxes around. Sometimes the system, try as it may to help special students, misses them. This case gives a realistic viewpoint of what can happen to children like Max. We do not blame the system; Max is not to blame; the parents tried; but in education we simply have to work harder to look at our modes of instruction. One comment was made by one of the teachers before Max was excluded, which we found interesting. She said that her responsibility was to teach. If the student did not want to learn then she had nothing to offer. That is probably true. We have since heard the statement many times from secondary teachers. For all of the dedicated teachers who take responsibility for students and walk that extra mile, too many do not, and then boys like Max drift into society and life with nowhere to go.

Max's case was depressing and discouraging. Many of the cases cited in our discussions have had good endings. Most of the children we work with are given exceptional assistance by teachers once they understand the needs of the child. But as we stated earlier, the information on how children develop, and teaching methodology, along with teacher training, have not grown together. Teaching methods are well behind the technology. For every situation in which we find teachers receptive and well-trained in today's technology, we find many others who are not. We cannot rely on universities and colleges to somehow encourage teachers to return for continuous training even though many fields, including medicine, do just that. Training will have to be done within the schools themselves. Yet, the cutback in funds from the federal government, the economic problems of schools, and the increasing demands by teachers for better working conditions, all make it difficult to deliver new technology. In the final chapter of this book we want to touch on the problems that we find confronting the schools. We want to point out how children, like those discussed here, are not getting an adequate education, and we want to list those special problems in curriculum today that create the children we have presented here.

Chapter 6
EDUCATIONAL IMPLICATIONS
AND RECOMMENDATIONS

THE former case studies demonstrate the realistic application of the concepts surrounding hemisphericity relative to educational concerns. We stated in the beginning that our concern is for how hemispheric difference affected learning and personality, and not for the more popular concept of how to improve right hemispheric or creative function. That is a concern and a worthwhile area of curriculum development, but the more pressing factors in hemisphericity are those that relate to children who do not learn well due to hemispheric difference.

In working with children with hemispheric difference, particularly those with high spatial and creative abilities, many important insights have been gained concerning how children learn, and the often devastating problems created by school curriculum when such insights are not put into practice in teaching. Of particular interest in our work has been the phenomenon of learning disabilities. Having worked in the field of learning disabilities since before it was even called learning disabilities, we are somewhat excited about the possibilities of hemispheric specialization.

The foregoing cases have demonstrated that the application of hemispheric theory with children is helpful, but it is not a unitary or holistic new theory of child development. Rather, hemispheric theory expands and supplements other aspects of learning theory. As the central nervous system matures we can see how development moves first through sensory and right hemispheric development to a more abstract and verbal, or left hemispheric function as the child learns.

148

Hemispheric concepts give a substantial basis to the notion that children learn best through experiential learning followed by more abstract learning. Through the differences in hemispheric development in various children, we can realize how some children must be taught in a more holistic and sensory mode, while still others must utilize a verbal process.

But the truly exciting aspects of hemispheric theory are the implications evident in the concepts that can be applied to all children. In this final discussion, we want to review some of the general concepts important to all children that are derived from our work with hemispherically different children.

The Motor Basis for Learning

In the field of learning disabilities much research and effort have been completed concerning the importance of perceptual motor development to later learning. Yet, much of the research in the field of learning disabilities remains contradictory concerning the importance of motor-perceptual foundations of learning. Most of such research has focused on a "digital" philosophy of development, i.e. the relationship of visual hand dominance to reading skill development. Such research does not take into account the matrix of interacting variables in child development, or learning skills in the educational environment.

The integration of perceptual motor abilities, significant right hemispheric involvement with the linguistic aspects of cognition, and left hemispheric development occur as a continuously interdependent process in learning. The recognition of body parts, and learning to move the physical system in predetermined and coordinated ways, produces internal imagery upon which time and space are integrated. For example, learning to recognize a series of written symbols, letters, and producing the sounds in sequence to "gestalt" the word, involves significant right hemispheric based notions of left-to-right space and moving one's attention across the line in a left-to-right fashion. This fluid and tremendously complex behavior involves linguistic interpretation, but it is reliant on the child's ability to consistently recognize and discriminate shapes, while also interpreting those shapes in an abstract cognitive function. This is an interhemispheric activity.

If the child becomes confused about right and left, linguistic interpretation is altered. The word "saw," is read as "was."

In written work the process becomes reliant to a significant degree on spatial function. Not only must the spatial system work in a consistent left-to-right fashion so that the linguistic interpretation is effective, now the spatial-motor system must produce fluid and automatic movements in the form of writing.

The difficulties produced by imbalance in the efficiency and development of the functions in either hemisphere with the other produces problems for the child. We are not concerned with arguing about whether the right or left hemisphere "truly" has lateralized specific functions, it is evident in the child's production of information that there is a breakdown in specific sorts of function. If he is confused in left-to-right orientation due to high creative function, or if there is confusion in the production of letter structure, there is a problem. The hemispheric concepts give us a way to look at specific processes while their origin is perhaps less critical. But with the concept of hemisphericity then, we have a model of development upon which to understand specific difficulties of the child.

Hemispheric Foundations of Language Processing

In the language area, specifically, the concept of hemisphericity has profound implications. As was just mentioned, spatial motor development is significant in providing a temporal orientation for language. But beyond that, the differences between how "cognition" is organized in the left hemisphere as opposed to the right hemisphere are vast.

Cognition, mediation of sensory information through higher mental function, is usually viewed as a verbal-abstract process. Seldom is the word cognition used in reference to nonverbal or creative function. This bias represents the ignorance of nonverbal function in the past, before concepts of hemisphericity were introduced. Slowly the notion of cognitive function in nonverbal processing is being revealed, but too few educators or psychologists really comprehend its importance. As we have stated in the case studies, psychologists and school personnel tend to view behavioral and learning analysis from a digital and left-brained viewpoint. They do not, in their own cognitive processing, utilize an integration of nonverbal and verbal function. How can they then recognize these important concepts in children? The case of Jerry, with a verbal score in language function in the retarded range and a creative nonverbal score in the gifted range, illustrates the problem quite well. The clinical psychologist made no reference to this difference other than the probability that it represented either brain dysfunction, emotional disturbance, or both. Such a difference indicates either a basic difference in neurological function and development internally, or, significant problems in learning and culture within the child's environment. In either case, the competency of neurological function is so different that integrated language and creative functions cannot be achieved. When the available operational systems, the left and right cerebral functions, are so different, the child will have to attempt to utilize the most competent system. Should that system happen to be the spatial-creative mode, then the child will organize his behavior and learning in a grossly different manner than if it were the reverse. The child with significantly higher verbal function can succeed in a verbal world but the spatial child will have problems.

Cognitive function within the nonverbal hemisphere, by the nature of its operational mode, will be very different than that of verbal cognitive function. Yet, the characteristics of so-called cognition are evident in nonverbal intelligence. Some of the important verbal cognitive functions are as follows:

1. Recall of sequential and related auditory-verbal information.
2. Classification, categorization, and recognition of remote verbal relationships. This is the so-called abstraction process.
3. Ability to view information from an objective and nonpersonal stance so that emotions and bias do not color perception.
4. The ability to make new associations between previously learned information and new experience.
5. The process of accommodating recently assimilated information into existing neuro-structure. This follows the recognition of remote associations and brings new information into the system by integrating it with its appropriate categories.

6. Transformations and temporalization — A most significant
cognitive function is that of being able to transform information internally into forms that do not now exist. This involves holding imagery of previously learned data in consciousness while manipulating and changing it to practice
alternate forms of it in the future. A significant aspect of
this function is that of organizing information and mental
operations into time and space changes.

These few examples illustrate the sort of thought processes
that are usually associated with so-called cognition. These processes have traditionally been in the realm of verbal abilities. Yet,
all of these functions are also part of nonverbal function. The
major difference between performing these cognitive functions
verbally and spatially is the mode of sensory data used. In verbal
functions the mode is representational, that is symbolic rather
than configurational. Verbal function utilizes abstractions while
nonverbal function uses imagery directly. Both processes are used
most efficiently in an integrated manner. But it is possible to perform the functions in either verbal or nonverbal ways. The exciting fact is that verbal function, abstraction, is dependent upon
spatial imagery function, and therefore higher level thought processes are usually an integrated verbal-spatial process, although
each can be performed separately. The visual imagery thinker and
the verbal thinker may come to very different conclusions about
a specific problem. It is through the integration of these two functions that allows efficient higher thought processing in cognition.

Without going further and getting into an esoteric discussion
of learning theory, these brief points are important to understand,
for the child with significant hemispheric difference will process
information in different yet complex ways. Hemispheric difference favoring either verbal or spatial function then can alter both
the child's performance on learning tasks and affect behavioral
characteristics.

In these two areas, spatial motor and language function, there
are important variables that affect the child's overall efficiency in
behavior and learning. Only when these differences are recognized
and the child's major mode of information processing analysed,
can we know how to teach him and how to assist him in managing

his behavior. Once the differences are recognized we can both teach to his style of processing, and/or attempt to improve the deficit process.

The following areas of developmental learning are those that commonly present problems for the child with high spatial abilities in the course of regular education. Most of these have been discussed throughout the case studies. A review here will assist the teacher in recognizing the needs of the spatial child and, through the process of instruction, assist the child in learning effectively. But there is an additional element in these specific instructional areas; *many* children would learn more efficiently if these general guidelines were followed. In essence, these areas compose a special list of needs for the spatial child, but there are many children who, though not high spatial children, would also benefit from these approaches.

Gross Motor Skills

If children can walk and run reasonably well, then it is assumed that they are developing adequately in large muscle function. But an adequate gross motor structure requires more than merely walking and running. While the gross motor functions, endurance, strength, and coordination are important, it is the later structure that is the key. Children today, particularly those in urban areas, though rural children may suffer also, do not seem to develop the keen awareness of kinesthetic feedback that allows more than just good balance and gross motor coordination. The establishment of good kinesthetic feedback and adequate gross motor function provides the internal reference for directionality, the awareness and projection of body parts, and dimensions into space.

Based on gross motor and kinesthetic function the child's awareness of directionality, and his orientation to left and right, up and down, front and rear, are also developed. This, of course, lays the basis for eventual fine motor and temporal orientation to left and right in educational activities. We have found that the high spatial child, with his uncertainty in hand dominance, is far worse off if he has poor kinesthetic skills as well. In fact, many children without high right hemispheric dominance have difficulty in directional orientation. But with the tendency toward avoiding directional dominance in the high spatial child, the additional deficit in kinesthetic skills makes the matter even worse.

The problem could be greatly alleviated if preschool and kindergarten programs would attend more to both gross motor and kinesthetic development. There is no lack of literature on activities for young children in this area. But a great barrier stands between helping children resolve these difficulties routinely, as part of curriculum, and the actual case in public schools. The barrier is the nearly myopic viewpoint educators too often have about physical education for young children. In today's schools, while there are many exceptions, physical education remains a sport-oriented program that often is not even taken seriously until fourth or fifth grade. Few schools have a developmental physical education program for children from kindergarten through third grade, which is precisely when they need it the most. In studies we have conducted with elementary teachers, they generally have little or no specific knowledge about what abilities are important in this area, or what activities would develop such abilities. A good program of developmental physical education given to young children for at least 30 minutes each day could do much toward assuring that all children develop the needed kinesthetic skills. Without the development of such skills the children are certain to have poor fine motor skills.

Fine Motor Skills and Learning Readiness

Following the basic gross motor, body concept, directionality and temporal-sequential organization, the child should learn to utilize his hands and fingers in fine movements that result in making basic forms and then letters. Here, without adequate gross motor and body concept ability, the child finds it difficult to relate fine motor movements to some internal reference such as left and right. As a result the child finds the small movements difficult to reproduce according to the angles and directions of the form or letter. The high spatial child, with his already confused directionality, finds it very difficult to move his hand in the proper direction to reproduce a square, and particularly a triangle. The vertical lines are the easiest for they require no special left-to-right orientation. Horizontal lines are no problem either in that he can begin at either side and move across the page. But later, which direction he moves will be important. The square and the triangle do produce problems for they require a number of movements in specific directions regardless of where he begins.

Thus, for the child with spatial-directional confusion such as the high right hemispheric child or the immature child, early fine motor exercises are difficult, and he will often avoid them. Obviously this will precipitate problems in making letters.

At this stage, in late preschool, four years of age, and early kindergarten, the teacher can recognize those children that are having difficulty with accuracy, directional orientation, endurance, size, and fluidity of movements. The problem will be obvious in the child's working behaviors and it will be obvious in his results. No special test need be given to see the problems the child is having. We cannot brush it off as immaturity either, for these children will continue to avoid those activities which are not fun or for which they feel failure. The teacher then, in kindergarten particularly, should address herself to these needs. This will involve a copious amount of practice, preferably on a blackboard until the children can master the movements. First, as always, we start with large movements on the blackboard and, while the child may have difficulty, he is continuously given much support and encouragement. If necessary he is given templates in the initial stages. This practice must continue, along with gross motor and balance activities if needed, until the child can reproduce the basic forms adequately. Again, any good reference on learning disabilities, and spatial motor and perceptual problems, provides the teacher with an abundance of specific exercises.

Finally, when the children are ready to begin letters, the level of difficulty increases tremendously, for now the child must combine language and fine motor movements. If the fine motor movements are not adequately developed, then this area will become particularly difficult.

The child has to remember the "name" and recall the structure. It is here that the problem in "automation," mentioned in the case studies, becomes evident and has its early and often innocuous beginning without the teacher's awareness. The right hemispheric child will tend to have difficulty recalling the correct name for a specific structure, or, recalling the structure mentally that goes with the correct name. This means that an inordinate amount of practice must be focused on these children or any child who is having such difficulty. These children must work on the blackboard until the letters are firmly established relative to structure. In that high spatial children often copy the letter without "thinking" of the name of the letter, we have to assure that the name is used every time they make the letter. Otherwise the child could just as well be copying Russian or Spanish, for after he is done he will not know what letters he has copied. This can be avoided by having the child say the letters as he makes them. Again, specific methodology is available in much of the literature and the teacher should develop a program from available information rather than simply following a preset curriculum for every child.

Early Reading Skills

Many of the cases cited in this book have illustrated time and time again that the high spatial child will tend to look at the whole word and use configuration or specific structural cues in early reading rather than phonetic orientation. It is not so much that phonetics cannot be learned but rather, as we have pointed out, they must be learned within a specific sequence in early reading skills. If a child is a high verbal child, then things work out pretty well, but in our experience more than 30 percent of any class of first graders will tend to be spatially oriented rather than verbally oriented.

The high spatial child, if he is taught phonetics, often becomes frustrated and has significant feelings of failure. This results in a negative attitude, not only toward reading, but toward school. The teacher becomes frustrated and the whole situation deteriorates rapidly before either the child or teacher understands the problem.

High spatial children should begin with many sight words, with word families, prefixes and suffixes, syllables, and compound sight words until they have a good basis for early reading. Then phonetics can be introduced, moving from the chunks to the

specific, from prefixes and suffixes to blends, and finally conso-
nants and vowels.

The teacher then must have a range of skills from language
experience to formal phonetics in her strategies of teaching reading. The first and second grades are critical and should be tied
together into a teaching unit rather than the practice of having
two distinct grade units for teaching.

Creative Writing

The term creative writing usually applies to those activities in
which the child makes up and writes his own stories. We want to
alter that definition somewhat for our purposes here.

Much of the children's work in school involves writing models
or writing whatever is correct according to a specific assignment.
Creative writing, commonly thought of as writing one's own
thoughts, should be much expanded in school programs. Further,
a child should not have to wait until he is able to write well until
this activity occurs. Creative writing involves a very significant
cognitive activity, it involves organizing one's thoughts and putting
them on paper in such a way that other people can understand
them. This involves the child's language and creative skills. It helps
the child learn to organize his thoughts and make decisions relative to sequence and outcome. It involves to some degree a great
number of the cognitive abilities mentioned earlier, except they
are in both verbal and creative functions. They must be integrated.

The highly creative child can often have problems in this area.
Even though he has a significant amount of creative imagery and
imagination available to him, he also has poor language skills and
difficulty in explaining and expressing his thoughts in a logical
and effective way.

Creative writing is used in language experience approaches to
reading. It is the creativeness which makes it a particularly valuable approach for high spatial and creative children. By stimu-
lating a child to organize his thoughts and encouraging his imagination, we are able to not only assist him in reading, but also in
improving his language organization. This is also why the creative
child often dislikes, and has so much difficulty with, phonetics.
Not only are the sounds hard to remember and organize, but the

stories do not make much sense either. The creative child tends to elaborate on the stories he hears and yet is unable to relate the elaboration to the teacher. By using language experience we enter into the child's world, his thoughts, and his imagination, and help him learn how to organize it so others can share his ideas.

For these reasons the high creative and spatial child should be encouraged to write creative stories. Of course, in the beginning their stories have to be verbal and simple and placed on paper for him. He can then read his own thoughts and this feedback assists in structuring his memory and organization.

Self-consciousness

Children come to us with all sorts of mental organizations and competencies in the nature of their specific conscious structure. One key word that is often used but not truly understood is "self-consciousness." Self-consciousness is typically viewed as relating to social values. We say a child is self-conscious, meaning shy or uncertain of self. We say that he should raise his self-consciousness, to become more responsible and aware of his own behavior, or in general simply ask that the child be more aware of his inner self. Self-consciousness differentiates between self orientation and directedness, and those activities in which a child may be driven to verbal or spatial activity which is undirected. The child engrossed in a computer game is a good example of being driven by some sort of mental activity in which there is a minimum, at the time, of self-consciousness. Even reading, a highly skilled task, at its most efficient level of processing, becomes a nonconscious activity. The digital and analog interaction of information processing, during highly efficient reading, causes the individual to become absorbed in the story and oblivious to the actual reading. This differs of course from technical reading in which the individual has to focus attention on the task of evaluation. But in reading for recreation the individual experiences the story and becomes a member of the drama.

If the teacher can understand that a child must *learn* to concentrate in order to become "involved" in so-called attention-related interaction, the nature of the child's attention or lack of it makes more sense. The child has to be taught and encouraged to develop increased ability in maintaining consciousness. In most cases we tend to perceive an individual in a holistic manner, assuming a somewhat integrated organization. In fact, we move from a conscious orientation to an involved information mode continuously. The child with poorly learned attention skills, with a poorly developed ·conscious orientation to self and behavior, and with significantly different efficiencies between hemispheric function, may have great difficulties in maintaining a conscious orientation to behavior.

The naturalistic child then often acts impulsively, without mediation of the events in his environment, in what seems to be a highly egocentric manner. Yet, in fact, the child may be unaware rather than egocentric. The teacher must realize that depending on all of these variables, the child may actually have difficulty maintaining control of the system, or orienting to the activities in the classroom. It is the teacher's responsibility then, to assist the child in orienting without disciplining him or making him feel badly about himself.

Teachers often tell us that children have to learn to accept responsibility. This of course, usually means that they feel the child is not behaving in ways acceptable or expected by them. But when we get such a statement we always ask how the child will learn such a thing? It is not something that will just happen. We have to help him organize his behavior. In a very real sense, this does mean help "him" organize his behavior or more aptly, gain control of the system, separate the behavior from "him." Often it does help to say "I love you, but your behavior is not acceptable." It is the inappropriateness of the action that the child must understand, not that there is something wrong with "him." This sounds silly to some people but it actually implies a deeper meaning than most of us are aware of neurologically. We are really trying to "raise" the child's consciousness so that he can control the tendencies and activity of the system.

All of this is extremely critical to the high spatial child for the system often responds somewhat automatically to situations, such as, a bird outside the window, slipping into fantasy upon hearing a descriptive phrase, laughing at something another child does during study period, or simply becoming lost while drawing a picture instead of working on arithmetic. The child with a high spatial competency often is less in control of his responses than is the efficient information processing computor that sits in his head.

The child with highly efficient verbal abilities often has no less of a problem than the spatial child. The highly verbal child who has been overly disciplined, who is super self-conscious, and consequently is constricted in his behavior, often over-controls behavioral responses. This child is unable to respond, he is neurotic about acceptance, fearful of being hurt, and constantly seeks acceptance, therefore making him unable to allow natural verbal or spatial-motor responses. The system actually does not develop well because the child's consciousness is so in control that learning does not occur.

Reflecting on this sort of relationship between behavior and consciousness is critical in accepting and understanding a child's behavior. Childhood learning is the process of both increasing the child's control and operation of the neurological system and, at the same time, increasing his self-awareness and/or consciousness. There are a few articles or materials currently available that apply hemispheric theory to behavior or that assist the teacher or parent in understanding these notions about a child's behavior.

If we understand the relationship between behavior, meaning what the system does as a consequence of mediation or its own natural or learned operations, and how the child develops self-consciousness, then management of learning and behavior is a different process conceptually. We do not simply say to a child, "Accept responsibility." We must assist him in doing so and realize that for some children the very structure of their neurology may make this more difficult than for other children, even though "he may" want to learn to do the acceptable thing. There are some guidelines that we use both in our own attitudes toward a child, and to assist him which are often helpful.

1. We accept that many children, though certainly not all, are unable in themselves to control all of their behavioral responses. We look for intent rather than merely at the behavior. In one case a child may strike another child intentionally because he wants something from the other child. In another case the child may

strike impulsively in a situation where action leads to action without mediation. The two situations require different responses, and pose for the teacher a problem in observation. She must look for intent beyond behavior. In the first case we may restrict or reprimand, in the second we may redirect and demonstrate.

2. The younger the child or the higher the spatial abilities, teaching requires more redirection, support, practice, and demonstration as opposed to merely giving verbal directions. In behavioral modification for example, we may give the child a small timer which serves the purpose of maintaining his attention consciously to acting in a specific manner for a period of time, as opposed to merely telling him to sit in his seat and work. We are eliciting his "conscious" control of his behavior through an external device to maintain attention. Through this supportive technique the child "practices" attention and effort. He works to control his, or more aptly, "its" response. Given time and reinforcement the child becomes more capable of control. It is for this reason that behavioral modification works, not merely that a reward is sought. The child learns mediation, he increases his own self-consciousness and control.

3. We give children much feedback about their behavior and we work toward getting the child to use language as a mediator of behavior. This is what socialization is all about. As the child matures, his self-consciousness and awareness increases and he becomes more capable of monitoring his own behavior. Language assists the child in temporal organization. He concentrates on sequence in time. Working on time-space relationships is part of the developmental process of maturity. Some children need much more help with this than others. Those with poor language, with poor verbal skills and awareness of time and sequence, will be at the mercy of the automatic responses of the spatial-motor system.

In this brief discussion we should realize that in the future there will be more concern for looking at child behavior from this newer viewpoint of hemispheric difference. Further, working with a child in order to instill more so-called responsibility is much more complicated than the mere matter of punishment or asking the child to be more responsible. It is not always the "child's" fault that he is impulsive or disorganized, that he chooses to play instead of work, or that he finds fantasy more alluring than mathematics.

The Future Ahead

We have attempted in our discussions here to point to a more rational approach to the problem of hemisphericity, and to encourage teachers and psychologists to look practically at this whole area of right and left brain function. We should see the reason for avoiding too much emphasis to the concept as a panacea for learning difficulties and yet, integrating the workable aspects of such a theory into everyday classroom teaching is important. There are two major movements in education that will provide an even greater change.

In the field of reading there is a movement called "learning styles" which encompasses much that has been said here relative to hemispheric or cognitive styles. The notion of looking at the child's learning style and then providing reading instruction in a manner consistent with his learning style is not new. But the field of learning disabilities and the hemisphericity research has provided a sound basis for looking at learning styles beyond the simple notion of measuring gross differences in visual, perceptual, language, auditory, and other integrities of central nervous system function.

This area of concern will occupy educator's attention for some time, in that presently those who are advocating the learning style approach have not yet assimilated much that was discovered about language processing during the learning disabilities phenomenon, let alone the more recent concepts of hemisphericity. But as the field of cognitive psychology, linquistic theories, hemispheric concepts, and increasing individualized approaches, all melt into educational theory, many changes will occur in education.

The second, and perhaps more profound movement is that of the computer "craze" which is presently sweeping education. School personnel are rushing into computer education at a rate that can be described as no less than a mania. But, as is so often the case, the technology of computer assisted and based education is far ahead of the ability and skill of educators to keep pace. The authors are also critically involved in developing the utilization of computer instruction, and the potential for assisting children through such technology will change education, as it will society, in ways that will alter the very foundation of instructional processes. The rate at which all of these changes are occurring is leaving much of professional education behind. It will be years before the smoke begins to clear and the difference between technology available to assist children, and the skill of educators to apply such technology is integrated. Schools can no longer depend upon the universities to provide the training needed for teachers in these new fields. It will require that the training of teachers be a continuous on-the-job process. We are in one of the most significant periods of change in education. We trust that the field of professional education will find itself capable of meeting the new challenges.

BIBLIOGRAPHY

Blakeslee, Thomas: *Right Brain; A New Understanding of the Unconscious Mind and It's Creative Powers*. Garden City, New York, Doubleday, 1980.

Bogen, J. E. and Bogen, C. M.: The Other Side of the Brain, III, the corpus callosum and creativity. *Bull Los Angeles Neurological Society, 34*: 191-220, 1969.

Brown, Mark: *Left Handed: Right Handed*. North Pomfret, VT, David and Charles, 1980.

Dimond, S. J.: Hemisphere function and word registration. *J Exp Psychol, 87*: 183-186, 1971.

Dimond, S. J. and Beaumont, J. C.: *Hemisphere Function in the Human Brain*. New York, Wiley, 1974.

Dimond, S. J. and Beaumont, J. C.: The use of two hemispheres to increase brain capacity. *Nature, 232*: 270-271, 1971.

Edwards, Betty: *Drawing on the Right Side of the Brain*. Los Angeles, J. P. Tarcher, Inc., 1979.

Fadely, J. and Hosler, V.: *Developmental Psychometrics*, Springfield, IL, Charles C Thomas, Publisher, 1980.

Fadely, J. and Hosler, V.: *Understanding the Alpha Child at Home and School: Left and Right Hemispheric Function in Relation to Personality and Learning*. Springfield, IL, Charles C Thomas, Publisher, 1979.

Fincher, Jack: *Origins and Consequences of Being Left Handed*. Putnum, New York, 1980.

Gazzaniga, M. S., Bogen, J. E. and Sperry, R. W.: Dyspraxia following division of the cerebral commissures. *Arch Neurol, 16*: 606-612, 1967.

Herron, Jeanie: *Neuropsychology of Left Handedness*. New York, Academic Press, 1980.

Hosler, V. and Fadely J.: *Holistic Mental Health for Tomorrow's Children*, Springfield, IL, Charles C Thomas, Publisher, 1981.

Hunter, M.: Right Brained Kids in Left Brained Schools. *Todays Education, 65*: 45-48, Nov-Dec, 1976.

Levy-Agresti, J. and Sperry, R. W.: Differential perceptual capabilities in the major and minor hemispheres. *Proc Natl Acad Sci USA, 61*: 1151, 1968.

Levy-Agresti, J. and Trevarthen, C.: Perceptual, semantic, and phonetic aspects of elementary language processes in split brain patients. *Brain, 100*: 105-108, 1977.

Macdonald, Critchley, and Henson, R. A.: *Music and The Brain*. London, William Heineman Medical Book Limited, 1977.

Ornstein, R. E.: *The Psychology of Consciousness*. New York, Grossman, 1976.

Ornstein, R. E.: *The Mind Field*. New York, PB 1976.

Penfield, W.: *The Mystery of the Mind: A Critical Study of Consciousness and the Human Brain*. Princeton, NJ, Princeton University Press, 1975.

Restak, Richard: *The Brain, The Last Frontier*. New York, Warner Books, 1980.

Sage, W.: The Split Brain Lab. *Human Behavior, 5*: 24 June 1976.

Sperry, R. W.: A modified concept of Consciousness. *Psychol Rev, 76*: 532-536, 1969.

Samples, B.: *The Metaphoric Mind*. Reading, MA, Addison Wesley Publishing Company, 1976.

Springer, Sally, and Deutsch, Georg.: *Left Brain-Right Brain*. San Francisco, Wm. H. Freeman, 1981.

Virshup, Evelyn: *Right Brain People in a Left Brain World*. Guild Pub of Tutors, 1978.

INDEX